'Your great aunts offer you their collected fa
treasure. "Open," they say, "it is yours now" -
book. With the magic word "Sesame" these t
of a uniquely compassionate culture, a form ̮. ̮̮̮
melded and seasoned in England over three decades. It is now yours.'

— *Craig San Roque, Jungian analyst, Northern Territory, Australia*

'An inspirational guide to the art of bringing myth alive through drama. Written with passionate feeling and lucid simplicity, this book is indispensable for professionals, and indeed anyone who loves stories and longs to explore them with others and dream them onwards together.'

— *Jules Cashford, Jungian analyst and mythologist, London*

'A luminous, hospitable welcome to the many years of the work of the Sesame Institute…how fortunate for therapists, teachers, storytellers, and all who seek and cherish the drama of authentic healing.'

— *Nancy Mellon MA, Psychotherapist and author, USA*

'A magnificent resource of key myths and fairytales. The authors generously impart their prodigious knowledge about the value and meanings of these ancient tales. The book is packed full of ideas and suggestions about how the stories can be taken into movement, voice, and enactment. Along with this the authors give their versions of the tales that have been most important in their work. A collection that is worth its weight in gold.'

— *Sally Pomme Clayton, performance storyteller and writer, UK*

'This book is a tribute of love, an indispensable handbook for therapists, and a treasury full of the archetypal wisdom of the human soul. Love shines through the whole volume — firstly for a deeply missed mentor and therapist of rare talent, who pioneered a unique way of working therapeutically with myth and story. There is love too for the work itself, and for that company of the soul, the band of Sesame-trained practitioners that has formed over the years. Finally there is the love of story and myth, which make up the book's exquisite treasure. Just whisper Open Sesame, and you will be greatly blessed with what pours forth from this dazzling source. The healing power of story is laid before us with a largesse that is the legacy of Sesame.'

— *Jim Fitzgerald, Jungian analyst, London*

DRAMATHERAPY *with* MYTH *and* FAIRYTALE

DRAMATHERAPY *with* MYTH *and* FAIRYTALE

THE GOLDEN STORIES OF SESAME

JENNY PEARSON, MARY SMAIL
AND PAT WATTS

FOREWORD BY ALIDA GERSIE

PHOTOGRAPHS BY CAMILLA JESSEL PANUFNIK

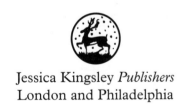

Jessica Kingsley *Publishers*
London and Philadelphia

The stories in this book have been retold, after having been received orally from a wide variety of tellers. As far as we are aware, all stories in the book (with the exception of two stories which originated within the Sesame community) are available in more than two versions in the public domain i.e. in published books or on the Internet. These are our versions.

Where we are particularly grateful to an author, we have put in a reference. We have also recommended, for further reading, a list of books which have influenced the authors in their thinking and writing about myths and fairytales.

First published in 2013
by Jessica Kingsley Publishers
73 Collier Street
London N1 9BE, UK
and
400 Market Street, Suite 400
Philadelphia, PA 19106, USA

www.jkp.com

Library of Congress Cataloging in Publication Data
Pearson, Jenny, 1936-
  Dramatherapy with myth and fairytale : the golden stories of Sesame / Jenny Pearson, Mary Smail, and
Pat Watts ; foreword by Alida Gersie.
    pages cm
  Includes bibliographical references and indexes.
  ISBN 978-1-84905-030-2 (alk. paper)
  1. Mythology--Therapeutic use. 2. Drama--Therapeutic use. 3. Fairy tales--Therapeutic use. 4. Psychotherapy. I. Smail, Mary. II. Watts, Pat. III. Title. IV. Title: Drama therapy with myth and fairy tale.
  RC489.M96P43 2013
  616.89'1653--dc23
                                    2013010971

British Library Cataloguing in Publication Data
A CIP catalogue record for this book is available from the British Library

ISBN 978 1 84905 030 2
eISBN 978 0 85700 438 3

Printed and bound in Great Britain

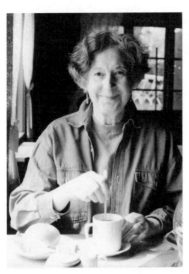

In Memory of Pat Watts
(1927–2011)

This book is lovingly dedicated to Pat Watts, Myths tutor, storyteller, colleague and friend. Pat's daughter Katie found the following words amongst Pat's papers:

> I would like to be remembered as someone whose mind was not entirely closed but open to new ideas and new views, with age you can feel you know the answers and that can be very irritating to other oldies (and) to people of all ages.
>
> There is a Japanese saying 'The warmth of the heart prevents the body from rusting.' This is a pleasing thought that that could be so. If not easily attainable at least something worth aiming for.
>
> I'd be pleased to be a good listener rather than someone full of answers and to be remembered in this way.
>
> Memory is not straightforward and often unpredictable. Sometimes people I have known in the past unexpectedly return maybe in a gesture or a tone of voice. Perhaps similarly I might be heard or seen again.

Pat Watts (October / November 2011)

Through the stories of this book, Pat is with us still. Her open-mindedness, her heart warmth, her quiet, still listening and twinkle of fun unexpectedly return as we tell, enact and are moved, as she was, by the healing wisdom of ancient story. We thank you, Pat, for your gift to Sesame.

Jenny Pearson and Mary Smail

Myths were not only stories told and poems sung, we tend to forget that they were embodied in ritual, in drama and dance and sculpture. The work of the Sesame Institute recaptures this ancient practice of embodiment and brings it to contemporary life.

James Hillman, 20 October 2008, in a letter to Mary Smail
after he spent a day at the Sesame Studio, then in Battersea, and
watched while 65 people enacted The Myth of Er

We're so engaged in doing things to achieve purposes of outer value that we forget that the inner value, the rapture that is associated with being alive, is what it's all about... Read myths. They teach you that you can turn inward, and you begin to get the message of the symbols... Myth helps to put you in touch with this experience of being alive.

Joseph Campbell, The Power of Myth, *pp.4–6*

We go to the myths not so much for what they mean as for our own meaning. Who am I? Why am I here? How can I live in accordance with reality? ... The myths never have a single meaning, once, for all and finished. They have something greater; they have meaning itself. If you hang a crystal sphere in the window it will give off light from all parts of itself. That is how the myths are; they have meaning for me, for you, and for everyone else. A true symbol always has this multisidedness. It has something to say to all who approach it.

P.L. Travers, What the Bee Knows, *p.13*

Acknowledgements

We would like to acknowledge and thank friends and colleagues for all they have contributed by way of time, thought and encouragement to this book, including our patient editor, Lisa Clark at JKP. Special thanks to those who gave permission for their anonymous feedback to be included and to those who participated in the studio enactment of *The Snow Queen* that was photographed by Camilla Jessel Panufnik. Our thanks to Camilla for her interest and generosity with pictures, to Alida Gersie, Jim Fitzgerald, and Pat's family for their continuing interest in the book and for the picture of Pat on page 7. Also, as ever, our thanks to Marian (Billy) Lindkvist for inspiration and encouragement. It feels appropriate that we acknowledge a debt to active sharing in the work of James Hillman, James Roose-Evans, Marion Woodman and the great storyteller, Duncan Williamson.

Contents

Foreword

Alida Gersie

When Jenny Pearson, Mary Smail and Pat Watts asked me to write a Foreword for a book with Sesame's[1] Golden Stories, I was thrilled. I had no doubt that this collection would be a great resource for numerous change-professionals. In my mind's eye I flashed back to an extraordinary story-workshop I attended under Pat Watts' leadership in London in the late 1970s. I was at the time a part-time lecturer in Comparative Mythology and the director of a new, arts-based community centre in the heart of one of Britain's most deprived housing estates. While both jobs drew deeply on my training as a dramatherapist and socio-cultural pedagogue I felt the need for some professional revitalisation. As such, the invitation to Pat's workshop came at the right time.

Our day began with some familiar movement and drama warm-ups that built up the group's energy and hunger for story. Then Pat invited us to find our own place in the room and prepare to listen to her tale. She recounted a legend from the San, or !Xam-Bushman, entitled 'The young man of the ancient race, who was carried off by a lion, when asleep in the field',[2] a version of which is included in this book under the title *The Lion, the Young Man and the Black Storm Tree* (see page 151).

The legend relates how a young man becomes unusually sleepy when out hunting. He lays down on account of it. As he sleeps a lion comes. It takes up the young man, drags him to a thornless, yellow-flowered zwart-storm tree and places him in its branches. Many intense events

---

1   Sesame is the name Marian Lindkvist gave to her pioneering work with drama and movement in therapy, soon after she began it in the 1960s. Based on the theories of Jung, Slade and Laban, to which she added her own Movement with Touch and Sound, the Sesame approach to dramatherapy has been taught as a course at Central School of Speech and Drama since 1986, and through Psyche and Soma, a two-year course for registered health professionals, since 2008.

2   For the first version of this story, see Bleek and Lloyd 1911.

later the lion bites the young man to death and the young man's heart-people kill the lion. 'And when the lion died, the man also lay dead; it also lay dead with the man.' Here Pat finished the story. Other tellers extend it with the formulaic ending: 'And there was peace.' However, Pat's telling lacked this apparent resolution. What happened after the deaths of both lion and hunter was left open.

As soon as Pat's words faded away, the group let out a collective sigh. We weren't too happy that she wanted this story to be the day's focus and that was hardly surprising. Each act of listening activates the listeners' individual preferences, hopes, fears and experiences, as well as their feelings about current or past socio-economic and environmental circumstances. Irrespective of the dynamics of our personal lives, we knew that racism was rife, and that unemployment, poverty and inter-group violence were depressingly common. The natural environment was also being destroyed at an alarming rate. One group-member spoke for all when he asked Pat to please give us a more 'optimistic' tale, but 'no' this was to be her story-offering, and moreover we were now going to enact it. In front of our eyes our easy-going facilitator transformed herself into a firm container of boundaries and expert manager of group-resistance. With the speed of the skilled drama-teacher she was, Pat instructed us to take a musical instrument, or some cloth that she had already placed around the room. We needed to choose the role of someone or something in the story (it didn't matter if our choices overlapped). While in role we should only use movement and sound. Words and direct speech had to be avoided.

Having said earlier that this was the first time she had met any of us, Pat took an informed risk. Playing someone else can be a very disturbing experience for people who are not comfortable in their own identity. Pat would have used the warm-ups to assess each person's internal and interpersonal balance, our ability to collaborate as a group as well as our capacity for containment, interaction and exploration. Her story-offering would have been based on this assessment, and not simply on her desire to tell the story, or on the fact that this was the story she had prepared. In fact the authors emphasise that such flexibility of story-choice is a key-component of working with Sesame's Golden Stories.

Hardly were we in role then, it was as if someone had turned a magic switch: our previously unenthusiastic group found itself immersed in the story's re-presentation. By mid afternoon we had enacted the legend three times, using, in addition to movement and sound, the occasional word or phrase during the last two enactments. In less than four hours I played the young man's mother; an 'invented' child who warned the villagers in vain that the lion was a shape-changing sorcerer who'd put a spell on the young man; and, together with two other group-members, the sturdy, long-lived yellow-flowered zwart-storm tree. After a brief tea-break Pat guided us through some excellent drama- and movement-exercises to bring us 'back to earth'.

During those few hours we experientially discovered that while story-enactment can provide insight, it rarely provides emotional or interpretative closure. Each enactment led us to modify our sense of the story's meanings. In each dramatisation we made different forms of contact with each other and with ourselves.[3] This taught us that, while the story's surface consisted of reported events, beneath it roiled our shifting gains and losses, our imaginings, hopes, fears and dreams, and how we made sense of our personal, social and collective histories. Scheub highlights that each story is told in at least four contexts: that of the story itself; that of other resonating stories; within the teller's personal history, experiences and emotions; and in that of the audience's personal histories, emotions and experiences.[4] Our three enactments made this multiplicity of story-resonances experientially manifest.

That day, as in every story-based Sesame session, there were two key types of performance. The first involved Pat's telling of the story to us as audience and collective witnesses to her performance. The second entailed the group's story-enactments with Pat as our sole witness. During each event we showed our emotions and hinted at our lived realities. Pat did so too – for example, her voice was audibly moved by one part of the story, and the group noticed this. If we'd been asked quickly to describe the day's observable events, this would have been easy: apart from some warm-ups and closure-exercises, it contained two types of story performance: ordinary storytelling and three story-enactments. If we had tried to describe how each of us made sense of these performative events, things would have quickly become much more complex, simply because these events were so clearly saturated with explicit and hidden personal meanings. There were bland statements that might have meant a lot to the speaker, as well as contradictions, and voiced or gestured expressions that were undoubtedly very unclear to one person and clear as daylight to another. The need for practitioners to engage with this

---

3   Pearson 1996.
4   Scheub 1998.

unavoidable struggle to articulate what happens in a session in order to move this work forward is movingly described in Chapter 4 in the book.

Back in the workshop's closing circle we took a little over an hour to share the feelings and thoughts, which, in Pat words 'had arisen from the enactments'.[5] Each person was able to contribute something, probably because Pat facilitated our reflective time with such compassion, skill, sense of fun and mastery. I remember saying that I'd loved the opportunity to enact the story three times. In each role I had expressed an important aspect of 'me'. The mother-role enabled me to convey that I was 'in real life' acquainted with grief. The child's role allowed me to explore some important questions around life, death and meaning. While 'being in the skin' of the yellow-flowered zwart-storm tree, together with two 'workshop-mates', put me in touch with how much it mattered to me that I felt close to myself, to other people *and* to the more-than-human-world. I also keenly listened to what other group-members shared. Much of this was private. From a dramatherapy-perspective the day's key healing processes were: play, attachment, joint attention, sharing, sympathy and empathy, identification, projection, witnessing and the creation of life–drama connections.[6]

From the perspective of the present, the memory of that workshop still gives me pleasure. It had so many effects. At a personal level the enactments reminded me that my early familiarity with loss and bereavement had not only granted me a vibrant resilience, but also a bone-felt awareness of the ecological interconnectedness of all that lives.[7] This influenced my subsequent research and writing. It also signalled the beginning of a fruitful professional relationship. I taught occasionally on the Sesame course. When, some years later, I became course-leader of the Postgraduate Diploma in Dramatherapy at Hertfordshire College of Art and Design in St. Albans, Pat directed the Sesame-training. Our collaboration, which included yearly shared teaching events, eventually culminated in the accreditation of the Sesame training by the British Association of Dramatherapists, and then, thanks to the work of many people, approval by the Health Professions Council and recognition by the Department of Health.

---

5   Watts 1992.
6   For in-depth discussion of the processes and their place in dramatherapy, see Gersie 1996 and Jones 1996.
7   For a story-based journey towards resilience, see Gersie and King 1990. For specific material on story-based journeys with and through bereavement, see Gersie 1991, 1992.

I decided to share my experience of Pat's workshop here because it says so much about the Sesame approach to storytelling and enactment described in this book. All Sesame practitioners, for example, retell their stories orally. Such storytelling imposes a certain economy of language on the story.[8] Oral tellers must choose specific words and phrases to give their stories a near poetic, rhythmic quality and highlight their structure. This enables the story to persist in memory and enhances the likelihood that it will be retold. Sesame's oral style of retelling is reflected in the style of the authors' versions of the tales.

Because Sesame practitioners do not work from verbatim memorisation of a written story-text, they must be skilled guardians (and, for that matter, transformers) of oral lore. They maintain their role as story-keepers by:

- frequently listening to stories and experiencing them in the telling

- creating informed relationships with stories that speak to them

- participating in story-enactments prior to telling a story for the purpose of enactment to clients or patients

- building up a repertoire of stories that is well-suited to their clients.

The authors insist that besides researching the stories' background, change-professionals who want to use these stories will also need to develop such oral telling/listening practices, so that they can 'discover other details which may feel equally as important or relevant to them' (see page 205). This 'searching and re-searching into the story' invariably yields surprises. Let me illustrate.

After hearing the Bushman legend in Pat's workshop I wanted to get to know it better prior to sharing it with my clients. My research then revealed that the 19th-century San-narrators, who gave Bleek this legend, were forcibly displaced from their ancestral lands and incarcerated on the notorious Robben Island.[9] Few inmates survived these slave-like conditions. I was aware that in such circumstances people everywhere quickly learn how to couch experiences and plans in allegorical or metaphoric terms. The 'hidden' language ensures that guards can't understand what they are really saying, while the inmates can express to each other what they feel or plan to do. This enhances

---

8   Ong 1982.
9   Bleek and Lloyd 1911.

their chances of survival. From this perspective the San-legend can also be read as a bitter allegory for the violent relationship between colonial occupiers and indigenous people. This reading of the story does of course not invalidate other understandings, such as Caldecott's take that this legend offers us a precise depiction of one man's entrance into the world of higher consciousness.[10]

In his popular book *Creative Storytelling*, Jack Zipes suggests that when trying to understand a traditional story's meaning the storyteller must face the fact that many such stories portray real occasions of abuse, abandonment, brutality and oppression.[11] Zipes notes that these stories' depiction of actual maltreatment deserves to be named, and that storytellers do ill-treated people a disservice if they treat the violence in the story as primarily a symbolic representation of a psychic struggle, and not as an experience-close representation of real events. This book's authors urge future tellers of their stories to attend both to symbolic and to representational aspects of their tales, in order thereby to enhance that which can be good in our relationship with ourselves, with other people and with the more-than-human-world. To illustrate what this might mean I want to offer one more take on our San-legend.

It is well known that, like other hunter-gatherers, San-hunters and lions closely cooperate when pursuing prey. Their relationship can in fact be described as a truly ecologically reciprocal, inter-species partnership. Until recently Bushmen would chase game that was too large for them to kill towards a familiar lion. When the lion killed the antelope, buffalo, dikdik or deer it invariably left some meat for its Bushman collaborators. They in turn left plenty of meat for a lion if they got to kill prey first. The Bushman–Lion relationship was in fact so close and mutually unthreatening that in a survey of 1500 Bushmen deaths over a period of more than 100 years only two were attributed to a lion, and one of these could be disputed. To indigenous people this legend might therefore also have been a productive teaching tale about the importance of staying truly alert to the dynamics of a key ecological relationship on which the survival of the !Xam-Bushman depends. And so does ours.

Even though the future of all of us depends on our timely recognition of this interconnectedness, a linkage that is exquisitely contained in this book's Golden Stories, the authors remind us that 'The myths and

---

10 For a socio-political analysis of San-folklore, see Buuck 2006. For an exposition of the argument that the story encapsulates 'the agony of awakening to a higher self', see Caldecott 1993.

11 Zipes 1995.

stories offer an experience which every participant is free to feel and interpret in his or her own way, according to how it feels in the doing. That way the story never loses its capacity to surprise' (see page 213). And indeed, the full acceptance of the wisdom contained in that reminder constitutes one of Sesame's Golden Moments.

Alida Gersie PhD
Dramatherapist, change-consultant and writer

Introduction

Jenny Pearson

This book began with a simple wish to gather, between covers, the stories that the three authors have come to trust in our practical work as dramatherapists, working with myth and fairytale. Our place of shared beginning 23 years ago was the crowded, higgledy-piggledy site of Central School of Speech and Drama in Swiss Cottage, North London, its studios and lecture rooms cantilevered every which way to accommodate all things theatrical on a relatively small land space. It was here that Mary and I spent our training year as students on the dramatherapy course known as 'Sesame', with Pat Watts as tutor in charge of a weekly session, awesomely called 'Myth'.

It is impossible to exaggerate Pat's importance within the culture of Sesame. The Myth element of the course was her creation. It remains a central experience of the training, the heart and soul of a way of working that draws on a diversity of disciplines to open up the experience of drama for people who would normally have nothing to do with it.

Pat was a drama teacher, initially teaching in schools and the Guildhall School of Music and Drama, who became interested in the power and beauty of myth and its role in the evolution of the human psyche when she trained as a counsellor and psychotherapist in the tradition of C.G. Jung. She created her first myth workshops at the Westminster Pastoral Foundation, the counselling and psychotherapy centre where she trained, then in Kensington. People who took part in those workshops still recall vivid insights that came to them when they entered the great myths in role. Her skill was to enable people with no experience of drama to step into the stories without self-consciousness and become part of them. As well as these myth enactments, she co-ordinated, with the Jungian analyst David Holt, a series of residential Shakespeare weekends at Hawkwood College in Gloucestershire. These were astonishing jamborees in which around 100 people were divided into five groups, each group working on one act of a chosen

Shakespeare play, and on the last morning all five acts (or something resembling them!) were presented in the big hall, in chronological order. Sounds like a recipe for chaos, but the combination of free expression and strong boundaries in the group sessions, facilitated by Pat and various carefully chosen colleagues and trainees, opened up a sharing that was orderly and by turns dramatic, funny and strangely moving. I don't remember why or how I came to choose the part of Horatio in Act V of *Hamlet*, but I will never forget how it felt to be given the role of storyteller by the dying Prince and be left on stage, after the carnage, to tell his story.

Pat's unique combination of resources made her an obvious choice as the first Myth tutor on a new training in drama and movement therapy, pioneered by Marian (Billy) Lindkvist in the 1960s and 1970s. The inspiration behind Billy's therapeutic venture was a dream: thereby hangs a story, drawing together the threads of drama, Jungian psychology and Laban's analysis of movement, to form the theoretical base of the Sesame training.

Billy herself discovered dance movement, drama and Jungian analysis at a very difficult time in her life when she was desperately seeking help with an autistic daughter. At that time, medical understanding of autism was in its infancy and she was spending a lot of time, with her daughter, trailing around hospitals, looking for help and a diagnosis. At the same time, in need of a creative outlet for herself, she joined a drama group at the City Literary Institute in London. She soon became happily absorbed in rehearsals and performance: she played Polly Garter in *Under Milk Wood* and Titchuba in *The Crucible*. The seed of her Sesame venture was sown when she heard the actress Dame Sybil Thorndyke reply to a radio interviewer's question, 'What is drama?' with the words 'Drama is psychology.' Directly after hearing this broadcast, she had a dream. In her dream she walked into a hospital ward and found the patients communicating with one another in a lively and meaningful way. Watching them, still in the dream, she recognised that they were doing drama.[1]

On waking, Billy knew that she was going to 'do drama with people'. With Ursula Nichol, her director from the City Lit, she set up the 'Kats' interactive mime and movement troupe, touring health centres nationwide. With another theatre director, Graham Suter, and a few actors, she organised a series of workshops, teaching occupational therapists to work with drama and movement. It was these workshops

---

1   Pearson 1996, p.52 and Lindvist 1998, pp.16–17.

that evolved into the full-time 'Sesame' training in 'the use of drama and movement in therapy' at Kingsway Princeton College in London, with Graham as its first Course Tutor. The course was named after the magic word from the story of 'Ali Baba and the Forty Thieves' in *The Arabian Nights*, in which the command 'Open Sesame!' opens up a cave where treasure is concealed. Even so, the magical power of drama is invoked to open up the inner world of imagination and connect people with their creative potential.

In setting up her training in drama and movement therapy, Billy Lindkvist had the courage and originality to act on her own experience as an intelligent, imaginative woman, struggling (as we all must) to make sense of her life. Having discovered the relevance of Jung's psychology through personal analysis she asked Molly Tuby, a distinguished Jungian analyst, to teach her students. Molly insisted that if the students were going to learn Jung's theories, they must experience Jungian therapy for themselves. Initially this took the form of an experiential group, conducted by Molly herself. Today's students are required to be in personal therapy throughout the training.

The third essential element in the Sesame course, recognising the therapeutic value of embodied experience in dance movement, also derived from Billy's personal experience. She describes in her own book a movement session with the Jungian therapist Audrey Wethered, in which she explored the inside of a cave and connected with the painful centre of her being.[2] She went on to work with autistic children in a hospital setting, developing her unique contribution to dramatherapy, which she called 'Movement with Touch and Sound'. Laban's Art of Movement and Lindkvist's Movement with Touch and Sound remain key components of the Sesame course at Central to this day, with dance movement explored by the students in weekly sessions throughout the academic year.

Billy's emphasis on the experiential was perhaps her strongest influence on the generations of dramatherapists who have emerged and continue to emerge from her Sesame training. It is a key to the authenticity and confidence that enables them to stand firmly on their own feet as therapists. Working on a session plan for clinical practice, she would turn questions back to the questioner, saying, 'Try it out yourself and see how it feels!' Then everyone would stop while the person turned an idea into action. It helped that Billy had the grace to

---

2   Lindkvist 1998, pp.9–10.

value other people's experience of a situation in the same way as she valued her own.

It was this basic trust in experience that led Billy to the four distinct theories that underpin her training for dramatherapists: a practical approach to drama, rooted in the theory and practice of Peter Slade (who himself taught at Kingsway Princeton, pointed out to Billy that her work was 'deeply psychological' and steered her towards Jung); the embodied experience of dance movement, underpinned by the movement analysis of Rudolph Laban;[3] an understanding, combined with personal experience, of Jung's depth psychology; and, of course, her own theory and practice of Movement with Touch and Sound.

It is not our intention to elaborate any further on the theoretical base of Sesame, which has been described in more detail in two earlier books.[4] But it does feel important to set our collection of *The Golden Stories of Sesame* in a historical context that does full justice to Pat Watts and her contribution in pioneering and teaching the Myth module, which lies at the very heart of the training.

Pat carried the experience of myth at the centre of her being, but she carried it lightly. Drama was her natural medium and she conveyed what she understood of myth through that medium, drawing people into it with effortless skill and holding the space in such a way that we were able to find a path into myth for ourselves. What she did provide, along with a playfulness that opened up an easy way into drama, was a reliable rigour in holding firm the boundaries within which our explorations were contained. Arriving late for sessions did not go down well.

Ritual is a necessary container for any deep work with a group and ritual needs time boundaries. Within that holding framework, there was great freedom for each one of us to find a real connection to the stories that, individually, we found meaningful. Myth is a subject about which it is all too easy to be grandiose, a temptation that P.L. Travers, the author of *Mary Poppins*, describes with a slightly self-conscious humility in her collection of essays on myth, with its beautiful title *What the Bee Knows*.[5] Pat did not make grand statements about myth, either. But, like Travers, she had an intuitive understanding of its relevance to our deepest experience. As Travers wrote in the same essay, 'whether

---

3   Laban 1980.
4   Pearson 1996; Lindkvist 1998.
5   Travers 1989.

we know it or not, we all...live in myth...as the egg yolk lives in its albumen'.[6]

Pat's deep knowledge and understanding of her subject was immediately obvious from the reading list she handed out at the beginning of the Sesame year. At the same time, I clearly remember her saying, 'Don't even try to read the books during the year. It's a reading list for the next ten years at least!' She encouraged us to research very thoroughly the individual myths that we each chose to present in our sessions. Otherwise, she kept our focus on approaching the stories through drama, tapping into their meaning by living them, playing with them and baring ourselves to the experience they offered. By this means, we encountered the myths much as people used to encounter them long ago, long before the stories got into books, when they first came into being out of the universal need to explore what it means to be human. Enacting myths was among the earliest forms of theatre, ritually performed to mark and celebrate landmarks in the human life cycle and the turning year. This is deep magic, something that C.G. Jung, Joseph Campbell, James Hillman and others have written about at length in connection with the evolution of the psyche. All this can be learnt from reading. But encountering myth through enactment is very different from reading about it. It's about entering into the story sharply, in the present, and experiencing it now.

Pat's skill was in setting up a situation in which this miracle could come about. I clearly remember arriving in the studio for our first Myth session on the Sesame course at Central, having no idea what we were in for. After the briefest of introductions, we were invited to walk around the space, to run, change direction, greet one another with a gesture and pass on. The experience was simply of being physically there, exploring, literally testing the ground with one's feet. Moving into a circle, we got into a conversation of gestures and movements, which felt a bit challenging at first but quickly became playful and, eventually, relaxing. There was a sense of beginning to recognise one another as present and real and of feeling accepted in a simple, ordinary way. At this point, standing in a circle, Pat asked us, in turn, what we were looking forward to most in the year ahead.

I was surprised, even shocked, to hear myself say that more than anything I looked forward to exploring dance movement. But I had signed up for the Sesame course from a wish to work with stories! Something in the early part of the session had reconnected me with

---

6   Travers 1989, p.12.

a deeply buried love of dance, something I had not felt since leaving South America and the ballet class I loved at the age of nine. This love of dance was a feeling I had lost and forgotten way back. For the first of many occasions in that Sesame training year, I found myself suddenly reconnected to a forgotten aspect of my being.

In that first Myth session there was an indefinable sense of magic in the air. At one point we sat in a circle on the floor and passed round a piece of paper, on which each person wrote a sentence of a story that began with the biblical phrase 'In the beginning'. The paper was folded over, like playing Consequences, so that the person writing couldn't see what the previous person had written. When it had gone round the circle, the paper was opened out and the 'story' was read aloud – a surreal collection of imaginings that sounded crazy. Somewhere in that collective jungle, there was an anteater. Read aloud formally, this motley text acquired something like dignity. No one protested when Pat invited us to enact it. The enactment had some very funny moments and a surreal quality, like group dreaming, which, in retrospect, prefigured something of the group that we became in the course of the year. The paper was ritually folded and put away, to be revisited at end of the course. I remember leaving the session with a sense of having begun to create our own authentic myth, at once hilarious and awesome.

I was reminded of that first Myth session when I came to read, in one of the books on Pat's list, Peter Brook' s evocation of the essence of drama. It is right there in the opening sentence of *The Empty Space*:

> I can take any empty space and call it a bare stage. A man walks across this empty space whilst someone else is watching him, and this is all that is needed for an act of theatre to be engaged.[7]

The effect had to do with alerting the imagination, that elusive aspect of us that jumps awake in the immediate present and becomes excited, in a forward-looking way. Something interesting is happening, something that concerns me. I want to be part of it! Peter Brook's 'act of theatre' is not created by a thought or a theory, but by a physical movement in a specific setting.

So it was in our Myth sessions. The basic elements from which they were shaped were drama, sound, movement and a sense of physically moving in space, contained within an agreed ritual. Into this space Pat would introduce a story, the 'script' for the session, but only when the

---

7   Brook 1968, p.11.

ground had been physically prepared and the group was ready to take over that script and turn it into action.

For the first term, Pat brought in a different myth or fairytale every week. The sessions always began with a few warm-ups, followed by something more imaginative that prefigured the story. Our part in these sessions was simply to soak up the experience of living the stories, in role, at the same time learning from this experience how to keep a session both contained and open for those taking part. We never left the studio without being thoroughly 'grounded' in the here and now, ready to engage with the world outside. In the second and third terms, we, the students, took over the role Pat had modelled for us, each in turn taking responsibility for a whole session. A schedule was drawn up, allowing time for each of us to choose and thoroughly research a myth or fairytale before offering it to the group with appropriate warm-ups and grounding, allowing time for discussion at the end. In this way, we were able to soak ourselves in the experience of myth for an entire academic year, with the privilege of bearing witness to those moments of self-discovery that so often come about when people step, however lightly, into a mythic role. We experienced how people can be drawn together by myth and fairytale, pulled by imagination on to the common ground of human experience. This sharing changed my own orientation towards other people in a way that was irreversible. In the course of the year other people became much less 'other'. Going on to many years of further training (in counselling and psychotherapy), that experience in the Sesame group has continued to be the ground I stand on when I work with people.

An important factor in this encounter with self and others in the Myth sessions was a quality that Pat herself brought to her work. She understood the importance of myth from the inside, not going on about it but simply making it available for us to discover it for ourselves. The most valuable thing I learnt from her was the art of stepping aside and making room for people to find their own way in. By physically entering the stories, we were able to absorb the experience they offered into our very bones. Pat was simply and reliably present while this happened, with a quiet presence and confidence that made it safe for us to take emotional risks.

I remember being overawed by Joseph Campbell's *Power of Myth* interviews when I watched them on video that year, feeling little connection with what he was saying. I was too near the beginning of my journey with myth. Recently, I returned to Joseph Campbell and read the same interviews in a book.[8] This time, after more than 20 years of working with myth as drama, it all felt familiar – more like 'Now I know what he is talking about. I've been there!'

Pat had 'been there', but she didn't say much about it, knowing that each of us has to make our own journey into myth, as the inner landscape to which it connects varies from person to person. While its symbolic language is universal, the resonances it sets up in those who engage with it inevitably vary, according to personal history.

When we had the idea, a few years back, of gathering the myths and fairytales that have proved consistently reliable in session work into a source book, my first thought was to ask Pat if she had her stories written down. Over the years, I had come to realise just how good those stories were. Pat had retired from Sesame and was by then wholeheartedly involved in her new creative work, as a painter of landscapes and abstracts. She replied vaguely, 'They are probably around somewhere, written on old envelopes.' My friend and once fellow student, Mary Smail, at that time Myth tutor on the Sesame course at Central as well as Director of the Sesame Institute, agreed to join in the project. The three of us met and began to make a collection of the myths and fairytales we had come to value as material for enactment.

Once the stories were written down, it became obvious that publishing them as a collection of stories in the simple, pared-down form required for enactment was not enough. Some explanation was needed of the fact that they lack the colour and lively effects that make for what is usually thought of as good storytelling. This realisation set us off on a new path towards offering some account of the processes involved in working with the stories in improvised drama.

We agreed to share this task between us, each focusing on one part of a typical Myth session. Pat took on the first part of the session, which usually consists of some kind of physical warm-up followed by a *bridge-in* exercise in anticipation of the story. I took on the central part, or *main event*, in which the story is told and enacted. And Mary agreed to focus on the final part of the session that *bridges out* from the enactment and the final *grounding* that prepares participants to return to the outside world.

Pat gathered up her stories quickly and efficiently and wrote a brief account of the first part of a session. She did not live to see our project come to fruition. To our great sorrow, our good friend and mentor in this work slipped away from the world just after Christmas 2011, celebrated and mourned by all who had the privilege and fun

---

8   Campbell and Moyers 1988.

of working with her. Her legacy remains fully alive at the heart of Sesame's work to this day, supported by some published writing on the subject of myth enactment[9] and her contributions to this book.

Mary and I were left with the task of bringing the book to completion. The loss of Pat's presence during its final stages has, paradoxically, opened up the way to a full acknowledgement of her contribution to Sesame, which her natural modesty would not have allowed as a living co-author. It has enabled us, sadly but rightly, to dedicate the book to her.

The brevity of her opening chapter in this book was something I tried, without success, to work on with her some time before her final illness. She was not unwilling, but she found it hard to recall much detail of a way of working that she had left behind some ten years earlier. The evidence of her new creative life was all around us, on the walls of her living room – another world of vibrant and beautiful colour that was enjoyably distracting.

Mary, who has been involved recently and intensively in Myth work, has augmented this chapter of Pat's with a coda of further warming-up and *bridging-in* exercises, some inherited from Pat and others collected or created in the course of her own considerable work with myth.

The pictures we have included in this book (after page 126) illustrate Sesame drama and movement in action and were taken during an enactment of *The Snow Queen*, led by Mary in a studio at Central, with a cast of graduates from the course. All gave their consent for photographs to be taken and for their subsequent publication.

The stories that Pat contributed appear alongside other stories from Mary and myself, in Part II of the book.

The stories are what the book is about. With just two exceptions, explained in context, they are all by the great author Anon. They are 'found' stories, not written stories, from different traditions around the world, which is why none of us have put our names to them. Great is their power and lineage.

Storytellers say that whenever we tell these stories, a line of previous storytellers stands behind us, going back through time to the people who first found the stories. Even so, in this little book, as well as the modest 12 stories that Pat wrote down, others from her repertoire have been set down by Mary or me. They are not our stories, but in truth they are not hers either. They belong to our shared heritage. Our thanks for their presence here goes back to Pat and, beyond her, to the

9   Watts 1992, p.38, 1995, p.27.

storytellers who gave them to us all. And our good wishes go forward to those who will give them new life in the future, as drama.

Finally, it feels important to state in this context that creating drama with myth and fairytale remains an integral part of Sesame's clinical work across a wide variety of settings. While in some settings the work of Sesame is primarily movement-based and stories are not appropriate, I have been amazed to discover just how widely they are used with many different groups of adults and children. Myths and fairytales are taken into prisons, hospitals, mental health settings, schools and centres for the elderly and people with learning disabilities, as well as being widely enacted by 'human potential' groups and workshops.

Selecting a story for a particular setting obviously needs a watchful eye to the needs of the group. At the same time, an experienced dramatherapist who knows a group well can often find it useful to sail close to the wind. Not everyone would see *Hansel and Gretel* as a suitable story for emotionally disturbed children! Yet it was this story that one group of very troubled children demanded again and again. Working with them, I remember the children's eager participation, mocking and pinching Mary as they followed her through the forest in her role as the wicked stepmother.

The Sesame tradition does not go in for 'menus', prescribing stories for particular client groups. Sessions are usually planned in advance, but it can often happen that something in the mood of a group will jog the therapist towards a story that suddenly feels like the right one on the day. If not a fairy tale, it could be a Greek myth, a Japanese *Noh* play or a Native American tale such as *The Boy who Lived with Bears*. The secret is for every therapist to have a rich repertoire of reliable stories that he/she feels comfortable with and a good working connection to the group (though such a connection takes time to build and there are many occasions, such as a new group or one in which members fluctuate, where this ideal situation does not arise!).

We offer our collection of tried and trusted stories for other dramatherapists to work with or, perhaps, to use as starting point, a model for finding different stories in the vast cauldron of myths and fairytales that is continually bubbling, worldwide. Reflecting on the Sesame approach, we have presented it in a manner that is experiential rather than academic, in the hope that our book will give readers a taste of the world of myth and fairytale as it can be lived through the medium of drama, and that others will be encouraged to step across the bridge that separates the purely verbal telling from the live experience of these ancient tales.

PART I

Working with Myth and Fairytale

Chapter 1

Getting into a Myth Session

Pat Watts

I have worked for many years with children and adults using fairytales and myths. As well as teaching on the Sesame course for the use of movement and drama in therapy, I have taken many workshops in the community.

People come to the session for a variety of reasons. Maybe they want to have the experience of working with a story, or perhaps they are looking for something they hope will be therapeutic. Whatever the reason, something is needed by way of an introduction to assist the group in working together on the story.

Myths are ancient stories which contain all human experience. The language of myth is image and symbol. In connecting with them, we can be surprised by the depth of feeling that is evoked. We can find joy and sorrow, embrace loss, find our ability to survive and create something we did not know was there for the making.

In coming together with others to enact myth, we are creating a special space. We cannot know what will happen. One person needs to be on the outside of the enactment to contain and assist the process of creativity. I will call this person the leader.

Although essentially working with improvisation, the leader needs to have chosen the myth with care, considering possible implications of the story and the effect it might have on the particular group. It is important that the leader does not take on a role but remains outside the action, though vigilant. Occasionally, it is necessary for the leader to step into the enactment (as briefly as possible to move the story on). This can sometimes be necessary when a group member becomes too identified with his or her role.

Before beginning work on the myth, the leader needs to place attention away from everyday preoccupations, worries or anxieties in order to give attention in a focused way. There is quite a skill in placing the attention in this way and sustaining it.

Depending on the nature of the group, members may know each other or be complete strangers to each other. Before beginning work on the enactment, it is important for the group to feel relaxed and ready for exploration.

It has been my experience that, although working with story, people can become more deeply involved if they do not use words. Instead, use voice sounds or basic instruments such as drum, cymbal or pipe. In fact, eventually a small group within the bigger one may choose to accompany the actions with sounds.

The first aim of the leader is to help the group become a creative entity, by becoming more aware of themselves in a positive way, open to each other and willing to take risks. To this end, I will offer a selection of possible introductory activities used to facilitate the group towards enacting the story.

1. Move around in the space, keeping as far as possible from others.

2. Move around in the space, keeping as near as possible to each other.

3. On a signal move quickly into a circle. Hold hands. Look at people standing on either side. Look at the group. Relinquish hands.

4. One at a time, move into the centre of the circle saying your name on a chosen rhythm. Everyone copy this. Go round the group in this way.

5. Select the name of one other. Repeat in the way it is introduced. Repeat your own name and movement.

6. Mirror partner, without using words.

7. Move into twos, A and B. A leads B with eyes closed on a journey in the space. Change over to B leading A with eyes closed. Talk about the experience to each other.

8. Without holding but using a hum or voice sound, A leads B on a journey. Change over to B leading A. Share this experience.

9. Work with a different partner. A to take a folded-up position, hold it. Eyes closed. B to open up A. A to allow this. Change over A to open up B. Discuss.

10. In a circle, leader to begin improvising on a sound and rhythm. Others join in. Suggest words – upset, relaxed, triumphant, sad and so on. Instruments can be used also.

At some point in the warm-up exercise I introduce movements or moods which are soon to be encountered in the myth enactment – for example, a dangerous journey, homecoming.

We come into the circle to hear the story, which to my mind is more living if it is told rather than read. The myth needs to be spoken clearly, simply with good energy. This is a time to be sure everyone is clear about the storyline and to select roles. Sometimes more than one person can improvise a character, in which case they must be sensitive to each other and work together. Some of the group may choose to work with the instruments and sit to one side of the main action.

Before enacting the myth, it is important everyone is clear about the story. Give time for the group to go over the sequence of events. Individuals choose their own roles.

The story needs to be enacted more than once. Each time, the group is offered time to share their experience and discuss.

The leader needs to be sensitively watchful. Sometimes when people are deeply affected they cannot talk about this at once but may be ready at the end of the session to share their feelings with the leader or one other. Always offer a space for this. Sometimes people find it impossible to put words to their experience at the time but quite some time later it may be possible for them to formulate their experience.

CODA: FURTHER EXAMPLES OF WARM-UPS

Mary Smail

THEME OF NAMES

Name echo

First person says their name three times. 'Emily. Emily, Emily.'
Group echo back three times using the same quality.
This goes round the circle.

Handling names

Explore your own hands moving and then find another pair of hands.
Introduce your hands to your partner's hands.
Each partner has a chance to lead the movement while the other mirrors (music is played for this).
Join with another pair and mirror the movement in fours.
To finish, each person outlines their name initial and offers their name to the others.

Name change

People stand in a circle.
Leader calls someone's name and changes place with them.
This person then calls a name and changes places.
Changing places can have different feeling qualities – for example, surprised, sad, searching, amused.
The speed of the game can be changed to fit the energy of the group.

Imaginary name

Each person in the circle offers their own name and a movement which the group mirrors back.

Think of an imaginary name for yourself and how that would make you move.

Introduce your imaginary name and a movement.

Come back to your own name. Does the movement of the imaginary name have anything to bring back to your name and movement? Share this round the circle.

Name dome

Individual comes into circle, says name and how they would like name said.

Group say the name back a few times.

This exercise can be sung or a sound used instead of a name.

MOVING ROUND THE ROOM

Own space

The space is your cocoon.

Play with far space and on the spot. Make shapes with the far and near space.

Play with near space, close enough to feel your body's heat.

Play between both of these spaces.

Where is your space today? Mark it out.

What is the colour, temperature, inside and out?

How does it look inside, outside?

Find your way to the door and have a look at the world outside.

Soon it will be time to explore there.

Purpose walk

Walking round room to music with strong beat.

Find the spaces in the room.

There is always room.

Don't strain to claim space.

Find the room that's there for you.

Being spontaneous

Say a word that comes into your head, round circle.

Make the first movement that comes to you, round circle.

Make a movement that empathises with the person before you.

Mood walk

Walk around the room confidently:

>   avoiding people

>   treating with disdain

>   shy but wanting contact

>   with a nervous giggle

>   seeing how close you can get without touching.

Speed it up or slow it down to fit the need of the group.

Walking and meeting

Explore paths in room.
Make contact with other hands – fingertip contact – and move on.
Group of hands come together.
Without words make a ritual.
Allow it to grow and blossom.
Allow it to fade and finish in stillness.

MISCELLANEOUS

Colour meditation

Think of a colour.
Feet full of energy – what colour?
Knees full of energy – what colour?
All body.
Find someone else. Show your colour/energy and see how your colours complement each other.

Standing on one leg

Two partners stand on one leg.
Without touching, what can you do to help your partner balance for as long as possible?
What helps you?
If you could lean on your partner, where would you want to be supported?

Short strings

Have half the number of strings for people in group (18 people –
nine strings).
Tangle strings together with tails out.
Each person finds a string end. Hold on and untangle.
Finds you a partner.

String tangle

Bring out a tangle of cloths, strings, ribbons.
Ask the group to 'make something' out of it.
Good before a creation myth.

Centre pot

Put into centre pot what you are bringing to session. Find an image/
sound.
Take out what you want. Find image/sound.
Ten minutes with partner to work out sound/movement sequence
with two discovered images.
Share with rest of group.

Chapter 2

Entering the World of Stories

Jenny Pearson

Since the earliest days of humankind, there has been a time at the end of the day when outward reality, with its physical and practical demands, gives way to a more inward focus, a time when people stop being busy and commune among themselves before retreating into the world of night, sleep and dreams. For a while, darkness is held at bay with man-made light, and for a few hours, traditionally, we enter a more reflective state of being.

This in-between world of evening has always been a time to gather with family and friends, a time to share food and stories. We share stories of the day, which lead on to stories of other days, other times. Eventually, we reach for a book, turn on the radio or TV and look for more fantastic material, the stories of once upon a time. Stories of imagination come into their own at a time of the evening when we feel the need for something different, something to lift us out of the humdrum world.

The fireside is the natural home for these stories. They come from a magic place beyond the fire. For centuries, before such stories were gathered into books, every village and most families had someone with a special skill for spinning them. Picture the scene. The evening meal is over and people are gathered round the fire. Someone picks up a musical instrument and plays a tune. They all sing a song. This is all the entertainment they have. And then someone turns to a visiting uncle or a grandparent sitting in the corner, a known keeper of tales, and says, 'Tell us a story!'

For many centuries the stories were carried in storytellers' heads, remembered and recreated with each telling, not word for word but by describing what happened as the story unfolded before the inward eye of the teller. Through the evocative magic of words, the people round the fire could see and become part of the scenes he described. Ben Haggarty, a contemporary storyteller, calls it 'poor man's cinema'.

The instrument of storytelling is the voice, primed by the eyes of a strong visual imagination. Skilful choice of words and resonance of tone bring the story scene to life. In that distant time, a good storyteller had a place of honour at the fireside. His presence, his unique energy and the atmosphere he created out of his very being were inseparable from the story in the minds of all who heard him. When they remembered the story in later life, they remembered the storyteller. Its transmission was personal.

So what does the tradition of fireside storytelling have to do with creating a drama session around myth in the 21st century? After half a lifetime of involvement in the current 'storytelling revival', combined with training and working as a Sesame dramatherapist, I always feel a deep connection between the two art forms. Essentially, this has to do with the depth and intensity of communication that arises between people who share the experience of a traditional story in a simple space, without the distraction of illustrations, props or technology.

The big difference between a story told to an audience and a story enacted as drama lies in the fundamental question of 'Who tells the story?' A storyteller recreates his imagined world for a relatively passive audience. He rings the changes of narrative, dialogue and description, bringing his audience under the spell of story through his unique music of words, imagery and rhythm. Laurens Van der Post called the art of the storytelling 'the literature of the living word'.[1]

Storytelling as literature is not what a dramatherapy group needs. In a drama session, the creative work is done by the participants. To enable this elaboration of the story to happen, it must be given to them in a simple, pared-down form. The details and inner dynamics of the story are left for the group to find in themselves, once they have entered it in role. That is why the stories in this book are presented very simply with only the essential details.

Live storytelling and story enactment share an interesting and, to me, exciting quality: unlike written stories, plays or films, they are unrepeatable. The same story may be retold many times in many places, but for each telling the storyteller relates the events in different words and with different resonances. In enactment, the differences are greater because every enactment, even of the same story, draws on the combined

---

1   Van der Post 1993.

imaginations and personalities of all the people involved in it. Each of them adds to the story according his or her unique experience, memory and style, as together they move through the story in role. As a result, no enactment is like another.

Being inwardly focused, both storytelling and enactment need to be kick-started by a deliberate act of transition, shifting people's focus away from the external world and making a space for imagination to find itself. Padraic Colum, the Irish poet, in his Introduction to the 1944 edition of *Grimm's Fairytales*, describes beautifully how, in the centuries before electricity and books, this transition came about naturally at nightfall. With the coming of darkness, 'A rhythm that was compulsive, fitted to daily tasks, waned, and a rhythm that was acquiescent, fitted to wishes, took its place.'[2] When the candles and fires were lit for the evening, the scene was set for stories. They belonged naturally to the rhythm of the night.

Today's storytellers are, of necessity, more deliberate in their scene setting. Often they light candles and create their own small spaces with screens, while for larger events they draw their audiences into tents and even theatres, consciously setting up a scene that will focus attention. As the audience arrives, the process of transition is helped along with small rituals, drawing them towards the threshold of a story. The Haitian call of *Crick?* tests an audience's readiness to listen. The audience, if they are ready to hear a story, will respond *Crack!* The call and response *Crick? Crack! Crick? Crack!* are repeated until the storyteller feels that the audience is really with him. This exchange has been widely adopted as a warming-up strategy by storytellers in the West.

When people arrive for a myth enactment, some physical activity is needed to enable them to set aside any thoughts and preoccupations they may have brought in with them and become present and ready to focus on a story, to become part of it. People who take part in drama sessions on a regular basis soon come to recognise the need for some clear process of transition. I remember an angry child I once worked with in a residential home who used to ask for a particular exercise at the beginning of sessions, knowing that it would steady his chronic restlessness and help him to enter into the story.

The process of getting a session underway has something in common with the separation rituals, described by anthropologists, preceding engagement in rites of passage. Their function is to separate participants

---

2   Colum 1944, p.vii.

from the familiar world and bring them into a *liminal* space where the mind feels free and psychological changes can happen. Creating such a space is essential for initiation rituals in which, for example, boys are separated from their mothers and taken away by elders of the tribe to undergo experiences from which they return with the status of men. There are, of course, huge differences between these, often fierce, tribal rituals and the more symbolic transformations that come about through myth work, but both need a *liminal* space for the experience to happen.[3]

The first part of a Sesame Myth session, in which this movement into *liminal* space occurs, has been written about in the previous chapter by Pat Watts. Pat was the quiet magician of this subtle time of transition. Her method was essentially physical and playful, encouraging people to let go of any doubts and fears, to relax and enjoy being present. What made it work so well was a quality of conviction and genuine playfulness that Pat herself brought to the task. She possessed the quiet certainty of an elder, in whose guiding presence it felt easy and fun to be a dramatherapist and make available to others the life-changing experience of myth enactment. Exploring myth in her presence was about discovering the power and wonder of the medium itself and finding, through her example, the confidence to contain whatever might happen by simply being there.

So the group is physically warmed up and primed for action. Paradoxically, they are now invited to sit in a circle for the story. There is an expectant stillness. Activity gives way to intense listening with attention focused on the voice that drops the story into the silence. The telling of the story matters. Although it is kept simple, it needs to be told with the conviction and authority that come from knowing it to be true. We are talking about the truth of *mythos*, the deep, symbolic truths of story as compared with the factual truth we look for in science and mathematics.

> Long ago, in a country far away, a king and queen lived in a castle overlooking the sea. They had land and riches in plenty, a stable full of horses, everything they could want, except for one thing. They had no children…

The story is pared down to the barest details of character and scene. The full telling of the story will happen later in the session, as the participants bring successive scenes to life, moving through them in

---

3   See Henderson 1967, pp.5–100.

role and discovering, within themselves, the human dynamics of their characters.

Myths and fairytales stand up well when they are told simply. The scenes and characters are easy to imagine because they chime with images and experiences that we all share. We may need to know if the king is rich or poor, the mountain accessible or made of glass, but mythic figures and landscapes have been with us since childhood, in stories and as lived experiences. Forest, mountain and sea have strong presences: they need only be mentioned to appear magically before us. When it comes to detail, each of us may imagine the scene a little differently, but we all know where we are. The words create a landscape and we are instantly caught up in the story as it unfolds outside clock time, a long way from the room where we are sitting.

The telling of the story is followed by a brief silence. Then the group is reminded of the characters, in turn. Does anyone feel drawn towards a role? Roles for the enactment are not assigned: they are simply offered. People are invited to choose. If one role attracts two or three people, it can be shared. There is no need to consider how this will affect an audience, as there is no audience beyond the rest of the group. The enactment is set up as something to be experienced, not performed.

A person with no experience of improvisation may find it hard to imagine stepping into a myth or a fairytale and performing it. In effect, it usually works out quite simply. Having consciously chosen a role, each person moves around the space in character, doing what the story dictates. If at any point the group loses track of the story, the facilitator will 'voice over' a sentence or two so that it gets going again. No one is required to do any 'acting', as such, but as the action gets underway it is not long before people find themselves living, breathing and feeling their parts. What may have begun hesitantly, even with a touch of embarrassment, lightens up and the story comes to life.

This is something we have all done as children, playing cops and robbers, hunter and hunted, doctors and patients, parents and children, or astronauts riding a rocket to the moon. All children imitate and play at those aspects of the adult world that catch their fancy. These spontaneous childhood dramas were researched extensively by the drama teacher Peter Slade, in playgrounds across Britain, forming the base of the unique approach to drama teaching that he describes in his book *Child Drama*. Slade relates how children at play will set up these enactments by common consent, taking on roles and entering, deliberately and consciously, into *The Land* of imagination to perform their 'story'. The world of the story becomes completely 'real' to them until it has been played out, when they will step out of it and go straight back to being their ordinary selves.[4]

Whether we remember anything of this after growing up, Slade's *Land* of dramatic play is familiar at a deep level of memory, rediscovered the moment we enter the land of myth in a drama. Billy Lindkvist recognised this connection when she set up her training for dramatherapists in the 1960s and she invited Slade to be a course tutor. His playground observations and the techniques evolved in his practical work with drama, based on the playground research, are firmly imbedded in the Sesame approach to dramatic improvisation, as it has been passed down through successive generations of trainees and tutors on the Sesame course. Although later, more sophisticated theories have been added over the years, there remains something vital and grounding in Slade's connection to this universal aspect of drama, which is particularly useful when setting up enactments with client groups in a clinical setting.

So people with no previous experience, having agreed to participate physically in a story, find themselves living it. The empty space transforms into the castle, forest or seashore where the action takes place. The dramatherapist's role is a neutral one, holding the space while people find their way through the story. The arena thus contained has much in common with Winnicott's 'potential space'.[5] In primitive terms, it is the space where a child feels sufficiently safe to play by himself in the presence of the mother. In this way, too, going back beyond the playground, the experience of a drama session can feel vaguely familiar. Suddenly, it becomes safe to drop one's habitual defences and be genuinely playful. To many people, the discovery that such a place can be found is immensely liberating and healing.

In setting up a space for an enactment to take place, clarity and decisiveness are required. The main locations of the story must be clearly designated before the action begins, so that the characters have a physical arena in which to locate and move through their story: a house or castle in this corner of the room, a forest over there, or whatever the story requires. With the essential characters cast and the main locations decided, freedom is then allowed for spontaneous

---

4   Slade 1954, p.47.
5   Winnicott 1971, p.47.

improvisation of minor roles and details. People can form doorways or boats, or spontaneously become trees, waves or fish in the sea, animals, incidental characters, a cloud or a bucket to be let down a well. Details of the story are available for anyone to elaborate, as imagination takes them, around the action.

A Sesame enactment is generally non-verbal, allowing the action to flow and not be held up by the struggle to remember words. If some words are clearly remembered and someone wants to speak them, that's fine. But, in general, communication is by movement, gesture and various forms of vocal sound. These can be expressive in many ways, using noises, vowels and consonants, or even improvised song. There may be outbursts of *gobbledygook*, as, for example, when Mrs Noah scolds her husband for telling her to go into the ark. Expressive movement may be accompanied by simple musical instruments. A collection of basic instruments, mainly percussion, is usually provided on the side of the acting space for people to accompany the action. This accompaniment is provided by participants who are not, at that moment, taking part in the story. The extent to which music comes into a myth enactment will depend partly on the style of the individual dramatherapist: most have a few instruments that they bring along to sessions. Some use recorded music in warm-ups, while others never do. The extent to which the instruments are played in a session often reflects the amount of attention given to them in the warm-up. Likewise, attention given to the elements of dance movement and voice in the warm-up will tend to influence the style of the enactment. The effect of warm-ups on the subsequent enactment is particularly noticeable when working with people who are new to the Sesame approach. An ongoing group will become increasingly richer and more versatile in the free use of the various modes of expression at their disposal.

Warming up is particularly important with regard to people using their voices. In Western cultures, we tend to be inhibited about making vocal sounds. Yet almost any group can be encouraged into playing quite freely with their voices if time and the right kind of energy are dedicated to this end. Acquiring skills and techniques that encourage people to free their voices has been a strong element in the Sesame training since the early days, when Pat Watts engaged the Voice Workshop pioneer Frankie Armstrong to come along regularly and work with the students. Frankie's enlivening approach to voice, often employing rhythms associated with manual labour such as hoeing and pounding wool, can get the most inhibited person experimenting with hollers and chants and 'mini mouth operas', preparing the way for very vocal dramas.

The universality of myths and fairytales is a royal road for people seeking aliveness and meaning, vital components of our life experience that are all too easily lost, not just through depression but under the ordinary pressures that beset people's lives. There is something in the very structure of traditional stories that makes them at once containing and trustworthy as a means of rediscovering our deepest selves within role. An inner prompting seems to draw people, more or less unconsciously, towards parts that connect with some hidden need. The moment I have chosen a role, I have begun to move away from my habitual self, becoming, as it were, an actor committed to my task. The experience in role is not about performance. It is closer to those improvisations that actors work with in the early stages of rehearsal, when discovering how it feels to be that particular character as the action unfolds. Gradually, the experience in role connects with my experience of being me. It is this that I explore, as I dream myself into the story. If I have opted for an angry role or a sad role, I may find myself in a context that allows some anger or sorrow of my own to find expression. Another role may open up surprising reserves of humour or joy.

What happens by way of insight and self-discovery through the act of entering a story in role is connected with the experience of embodying, as compared with thinking about, emotional states. Winnicott, through his work with children, was very clear about the close connection between bodily experience and the 'true self', a feeling of authenticity without which we cannot be creative or feel real. He noted that:

> The true self is bound up with bodily aliveness. It comes from the aliveness of the body tissues and the working of the body functions, including the heart's action and the breathing.[6]

The activation of this connection to the body and accompanying sense of authenticity is a vital part of Sesame's 'oblique approach' when working with drama in clinical settings. What begins as 'Let's pretend' can quickly move into experiences that connect, however fleetingly, with an elusive 'true self', which is vulnerable and habitually hidden behind a mask or *persona*, the official and recognisable self that we present to the world. The potentially risky encounter with the 'true self' is contained and hidden from view when it takes place in role.

---

6   Winnicott 1960, p.148.

The 'as if' element in drama acts as a safeguard against the danger of stripping away a person's protective mask or 'false self' which, as Winnicott also pointed out, is a necessary guardian self, protecting the vulnerable 'true self' from impingement and hurt.[7] Paradoxically, being in role simultaneously reveals and protects, within a dramatic convention that is contained by the ritual of careful de-roling once an enactment is over. The actor steps away from the role, away from the story world and the feelings it has aroused, and reconnects with his or her ordinary self, ready to return to the world outside the studio. The de-roling process bears some similarity to the Davis escape hatch that helps deep-sea divers to surface safely from the physical pressures of the deep.

C.G. Jung observed how myths and fairytales engage with our deepest psychological concerns, which is another reason why the gods, goddesses, heroes and heroines of myth and the more quirky, person-sized inhabitants of the fairytales have a familiar quality to which we can relate.[8] They embody states of being that most of us have experienced in the ordinary struggles of our lives. Entering into the stories, we engage playfully, at one remove, in adventures that resonate with our strongest fears, ambitions and longings. In Jung's terminology, the figures of myth give symbolic form to the *archetypes* of human nature.

These are powerful stories. They have lasted through the centuries because people have found them consistently meaningful and therefore worthy of being repeatedly passed on. They are the means by which our ancestors reflected on the meaning of things and educated their children, aware that story has a shape and a magic that will draw people in and be remembered. The full magic of narrative is that it creates a kind of learning from experience which is invigorating, as compared with the oppressive finger-wagging of authority, which many of us are inclined to reject. You are invited in, to stand alongside the *dramatis personae* of a story, to live their adventures and draw your own conclusions from the experience.

Finding wisdom or insight through a myth or fairytale enactment has something in common with learning from a dream. The dream feels real when it is happening. Then we wake up and ask ourselves, or a trusted other, 'I wonder what that was about? Why did I dream it? What does it say about my life now?' The personal significance of a

---

7   Winnicott 1960, pp.46–47.
8   See Jung 1956/1967, 1968/1991.

dream can't be looked up in a reference book. It is a matter of staying with the experience of the symbolic world and letting it speak, in its own way, within the context of the life we are living. The same applies to those insights that can come to us indirectly out of the experience of myth enactment. What remains of the experience in role can sometimes surface quite graphically hours, days, months or even years later, like the memory of a dream. And then comes the feeling of 'Oh, now I understand why that moment in the story felt so important!'

The great myths of the world all began as ways of looking at the big questions about life and its origins, to which there are no obvious answers. In some earlier cultures, the myths were staged as ritual theatre, with particular ones being performed to mark the seasons or stages in the human life cycle.

In ancient Greece, the myth of *Persephone and Demeter* was regularly enacted in the Eleusinian mysteries.[9] By a nice coincidence, a group of sixth formers became so excited about Stanley Kramer's new translation of the Sumerian story *Inanna*[10] in the 1980s that they decided to stage a performance of it for the Edinburgh Festival. They called their company Initiation Theatre. It was not until they were about to start rehearsals that a Sumerian scholar told them it had probably been performed as an initiation ritual 4000 years ago! Clearly they had tapped into an archetypal vein in their choice of script. This overlap of the personal and the mythological is well documented by Joseph Campbell, summarised by his statement that 'The myth is the public dream and the dream is the private myth.'[11]

The *dramatis personae* of myth are gods and goddesses, or legendary heroes and heroines whose deeds have raised them to a godlike status. All human societies have had myths about how the world, or the human race, began. Fairytales explore similar themes, but the manner of their exploration is not so stark, with playful concessions to humour and absurdity. The *dramatis personae* of fairytale are not gods and goddesses, but people of every rank, with a supporting cast of talking animals and supernatural beings. Not as ancient as the great myths, their source is closer to the domestic and to the imaginative world of childhood. This makes them in no way inferior. On the contrary, they have a charm that draws people in and a rhythm that is unobtrusively comforting. The Jungian analyst Alan McGlashan writes of 'the mysterious golden light

---

9   See Jung and Kerenyi 1941, pp.162–183.
10   Wolkstein and Kramer 1983.
11   Campbell and Moyers 1988, p.40.

that shines through myth and fairytale', observing how this quality of 'translucence' is often experienced by ordinary people in exceptional moments of our lives: 'in the first days of overwhelming love, in the final moments of overwhelming peril, in the presence of new life, and sometimes on the unheralded news of death'.[12]

Enacting myths and fairytales as part of a group, not for public performance but for the experience itself, is a form of sharing that stands outside the usual mores of our sophisticated Western society. It is closer to the ways of older and more primitive cultures, where song, dance and storytelling are taken for granted as activities in which everyone takes part. Out of this fact arise questions about why we, in the Sesame community, set up this kind of session work, and for whom?

I have already written of our founder's experience with drama and her recognition of its therapeutic value and how, with Peter Slade, she went on to develop the Sesame approach. Myth and fairytale were found to be ideal material for drama for many reasons: they are accessible, they are easy to remember and they have a resonance that is profound. Sesame dramatherapists use them in session work right across the range of clinical settings, from children's groups to the elderly, from people with learning disabilities to mental health wards and day centres, schools and prisons. I have memories of a small boy who worked through his rage against the world and emerged with an impressive sense of self, through many enactments of a story about three strong women training a Sumi warrior. There was a violent prisoner who initially found myth sessions hilarious, but came to value them after discovering and confronting his frightened self in a role. A schizophrenic man, who sometimes believed himself to be an alarming Old Testament character, was able to move quite sanely in and out of role when he chose, in a drama session, to play the part of King Midas. On this occasion he was not acting crazy, but simply acting.

Claire Schrader, in her book *Ritual Theatre*, writes movingly of what can be achieved by practising myth enactment on a regular basis with a committed 'human potential' group.[13] The continuity she established with her *myth-a-drama* groups clearly created an ideal situation in which to deepen the experience that myth enactment offers. A committed, ongoing group has time to develop a wide range of dramatic expression as well as a good level of trust. Indeed, it is the privilege of the Sesame

---

12 McGlashan 1988, pp.10–11.
13 Schrader 2012, pp.94–91.

training group to have such an experience on a weekly basis over a whole academic year.

Clinical practice, with its ups and downs, cannot offer anything like these ideal conditions, with the dramatherapist coming in week by week and groups whose membership is often fragmented and discontinuous. Nevertheless, myth has a way of getting through to people once they encounter it. Those who get it and return for more can surprise us with the creative use they make of it.

As ever, the way that myth is presented and the warm-up activities that precede it are the key. Hardest of all is a one-off session or a first session in a clinical placement. Yet in these situations the Sesame approach is fundamentally the same — that is, beginning with a warm-up and *bridge-in* appropriate to the group, so that people feel safe and become interested in what is going on, at which point they may be ready for some kind of experience in *liminal* space. Working with myth may not feel appropriate in a first session. Sometimes it is better to get to know a group over a session or two, staying orientated towards movement until they feel ready to focus on a story. And there are settings and client groups in which myth work is not an option, in which it is more appropriate to work with some other creative forms such as Laban-based movement[14] and Lindkvist's Movement with Touch and Sound.[15]

Coming out of a myth enactment, there can be a strong sense of having inhabited a different order of reality, not unlike a dream. The end of the story may have been experienced as cathartic, producing a sense of resolution and a kind of relief. Sometimes it can feel strangely sad or beautiful or distressing. Whatever the experience, the story is over. Action yields to stillness. The group returns to the circle and there is brief period of reflection. Is there anything that anyone wants to say?

People emerging from an enactment often want to share something of what they have felt and experienced within the story. The facilitator's role here is strictly neutral. It is axiomatic to the Sesame approach that no comment or interpretation of the material is offered. Respect for the individual's experience within the art form is felt to be the key to working within the symbolic frame of myth and fairytale. The experience in role can go deep and the images that remain in the mind afterwards carry a charge. Time and respect may be needed for the meaning and relevance of the experience to become apparent.

---

14 See Pearson 1996, Chapter 7.
15 See Pearson 1996, Chapters 9, 10, 21, 23 and 24.

After the story, the space is opened up for people to say whatever they want to say. This may or may not lead to personal revelations and sharing of thoughts. It can happen that a sense of completeness and peace descends and nobody wants to talk, which is fine. More often, the story enactment will have stirred up feelings and questions and it can be helpful for these to be voiced in the group. Someone may want to re-enact part of the story, which is fine. Responding sensitively to reactions in the time following an enactment is a vital part of the therapist's holding role. At the same time, care is taken not to let personal issues take over from the experience the group has shared.

The time of shared thoughts concludes the *main event*, which is the name given to this part of the session where the story is lived in *liminal* space. Just as this space was carefully and ritually entered at the beginning of the session, this movement has now to be reversed. There needs to be a clear exit from the dream world of story, returning to a state of mind and body in which people feel like themselves again, ready to take up their lives in the world outside the acting space.

The first step in this direction is to de-role, a procedure that requires sensitive handling, as there may be feelings of attachment to the characters in the story. The simplest de-roling ritual can consist of the actors ritually peeling off their roles and placing them, like garments, outside the circle. Time may then be given to brushing one another down, flicking off any remaining traces of the part that may be clinging to the person, the face, the hair, the feet of another participant. This familiar ritual can be amusing, but allowance has to be made for the possibility that the person feels attached to his or her part and may find this action jarring. As with every aspect of session work, dramatherapists vary in their repertoires for making sure that people are no longer identified with the roles they have been playing. It can be enjoyable for the group to stand in two opposite lines and form a tunnel through which everyone passes in turn, being thoroughly patted and brushed down as they go. De-roling comes up against interesting resistances. Particularly, I have noticed, people love being cows. At the end of the longest, most thorough de-roling tunnel, two cows from an enactment of *The Star Woman* were still moo-ing. However, the humour of the situation did the trick, breaking the imaginative hold of the story so that they were safely back in their own human skins before going home.

The process of bringing a session to its conclusion, separating the participants from the hold of the story and at the same time enabling them to take its treasure back with them across the bridge into the real world, is a task as delicate and subtle as the warm-up. My friend and colleague Mary Smail, who was Myth tutor on the Sesame course at Central for nine years, describes this concluding part of the session in the chapter that follows.

Chapter 3

Entering and Leaving the Place of Myth

Mary Smail

Question: What does the image of a bridge evoke for you?

A bridge...

Spans a gap between two places

Connects two pieces of land and creates a link between separate spaces

Provides a crossing between two points

Sweeps from one place of safety to another place of safety, moving over some lower, more risky terrain

A bridge is...

A structure that has been traversed many times and a safe connection, which is sturdy enough to enable the 'traveller' to go over without really being aware that they have done so

While it links across from one place to another, it is also a place in itself which aids someone to get to another place, space or state which, without the bridge, would be completely unconnected

The place of 'in between', somewhere perhaps where you are more linked with the space or air rather than 'earth' or ground.

(Response fragments from Sesame dramatherapists)

The terms *bridge in* and *bridge out* are familiar in the language of Sesame drama and movement therapists; indeed, all dramatherapy trainings take care over teaching their students to recognise and account for the imaginal pathway between outward reality and the symbolic world that dramatherapy employs as its royal road to well-being. This chapter will visit the idea of bridge as a metaphor for this path, allowing us to consider the connection between the inner and the outer worlds in the context of a Sesame therapy session. It will look at what we mean when we use the term *bridge*, and ask questions about the landscape these bridges span. It will address some of the practical conditions for good bridge travelling, and think about trust as a core condition for the emergent story, which consistently arrives when the external environment is attentive to the inner health-maker or teacher within.

It will also consider the obstacles that client and therapist encounter when they perceive and stand alongside the non-verbal content of the place at the interior side of the bridge, and consider how this is related to more verbal forms of therapy. How do we find the means to communicate the healing potential of the imaginal world to those who prefer to work from a place which draws its vocabulary from a base of knowledge revealed through the spoken word? There are many ways to think and communicate one's thoughts. The therapist has a responsibility to bypass the person's shyness by finding vibrant language that does not limit the inner process or bend it out of shape by superimposing an academic or scientific form. To have the confidence to speak with authority for psyche-soul in her own terms, and to discuss and write of this in real, hands-on language, is the challenge posed by the exterior land on the other side of the bridge. It is a task at which many struggle and fail. Robert Romanyshyn talks of this in his article 'The Wounded Researcher':

> We are called to build as best we can an epistemology that is ethical, reflexive, therapeutic, response-able, and perhaps even redemptive, a way of knowing that allows soul to recall what mind would forget, regard what it would ignore, and care for what it would neglect.[1]

Winnie-the-Pooh echoes something of the same idea:

> 'Rabbit's clever,' said Pooh thoughtfully.
>
> 'Yes,' said Piglet, 'Rabbit's clever.'
>
> 'And he has Brain.'
>
> 'Yes', said Piglet. 'Rabbit has Brain.'
>
> There was a long silence.

---

1   Romanyshyn 2006, p.38.

'I suppose,' said Pooh, 'that that's why he never understands anything.'[2]

The style of understanding intentionally used in this chapter has a *patchwork* feel, representing the oblique and non-linear way that the psyche uses words to bridge story resources back over into the world of the everyday. These image strands come into being through a process that I call *half-formed articulation*. They have to be stitched together to make logical sense, but we will come to this later.

I have been enabled by the help of 30 Sesame therapists who were invited to respond to seven questions.

1. What does the image of a bridge evoke for you?

2. What do you understand by the term *bridge out* in a dramatherapy session?

3. Can you describe a personal image, feeling, insight or thought which emerged from a story enactment through the *bridging-out* process?

4. In your work with others, could you share a time where the *bridge out* has provided a moment of connection or insight for someone?

5. How did you become aware of this?

6. Is the above what you would call, in Sesame shorthand, a golden moment?

7. What do you understand by the term 'reflective processing' as a means of synthesising the experience of symbol and metaphor back into thinking, words and making life changes?

Sections or *patches* created from their answers are sewn into what follows, in an attempt to represent the soul-friendly way of returning image to word as random fragments – parts of a whole. I hope this will allow the reader to think imaginatively when accounting for the *bridging* process in her own experience and practice, learning to trust the indirect image which is the first fruit of depth thinking. I am calling the active part of the unconscious – the non-sense author who translates and publishes the new, emergent story – the *psyche-soul*. I will say more about this later.

---

2   Milne 1928, p.127.

Conscious and unconscious, a bridge apart

Kharis Dekker, a Sesame practitioner, in her paper *A Door that is a Bridge*[3] writes about story and the *bridging* concept:

> Myths and legends as symbolic stories are a bridge between consciousness and the unconscious. The bridge is a two-way bridge. The conscious mind as the 'I', the ego personality, the conscious me, can approach the unconscious via this bridge... However, the unconscious can also be active enough to cross the bridge towards the direction of consciousness.

> Consciousness and unconsciousness are complex ideas to which philosophers, theorists and schools of therapy each attach a particular meaning and construct. These two words are therefore ambiguous as they have differing interpretations within each discipline and approach. A working definition of the conscious and unconscious self in a Sesame session might help us here.

> Personal consciousness is the 'outside I', consisting of what the individual knows or keeps in mind about herself. It is everything that involves the functions and conditions of the client's lived or outer story. It is the *awareness* from which we present ourselves, relate and respond to other people and the environment in which we live. Consciousness is all that we know and everything that can be remembered or recollected. It is the starting point of a Sesame session and the place in which one pillar of the bridge is firmly planted.

> The unconscious part of the personality needs to be described in an ordinary way, one which a session user can recognise. In common parlance, it might be known as something inside me, a deeper place, or the dream world. Freud and Jung are the great Fathers of thoughts around the design and nature of the unconscious in therapy, but a simple summing up of the inner world is offered by Michael Kearney, a physician who works imaginatively with terminally ill patients. He writes of the surface mind as the outer part of the personality, and goes on to describe the deep mind and the deep centre which lie underneath.

> > The deep-mind is the intuitive aspect of the mind. It is intimately connected to the emotions and the physical body. Its vocabulary

---

3   Dekker 1998, p.2.

is image, dream, symbol and myth… While it is the underworld of the unconscious and basement area where old hurts, painful memories live, the deep mind is also the location for great inner resources and childlike spontaneity.

The deep-centre is the core of our being. It corresponds to what Jung calls the Self and is closely linked to what is universally known as Spirit. It is the royal ruler in the depths of the psyche.[4]

I name these terms when working with clients and students, and find that when people feel safe enough in their conscious self, once they realise that the conditions of a Sesame session intend affirmation rather than judgment, then defenses, or held positions, gradually soften. There is a slowing down, a breathing space, and time to befriend the images of the deep mind and the even deeper centre. This naming is a delicate task. If laboured, it could be heard as having an evangelical or devout push, which is clearly counter-therapeutic in a culture which has become phobic about religion, often with good cause. When the therapist speaks obliquely of this place, through a story metaphor, she is dropping a hint that affirms the possibility of 'something inside so strong' as the song says, something that is wise and available and knows what needs to happen next. The Ali Baba story with its magic words 'Open Sesame' alludes to this when it tells of a locked away treasure which, when you are strong enough to enter the cave, will reward you. Edward Edinger sums up this process, '…when one pays attention to the unconscious, the unconscious is likely to show some kindness to the ego that does so'.[5]

Bridges and archetypes

Before we go into the practicalities of how to create a *bridge in* or a *bridge out*, we need to add one other idea to that of *deep mind* and *deep centre*, and introduce the energy and liveliness of Jung's *archetypes* in the work of embodying traditional stories.

Sesame works from a strong belief that everyone has inner resources which may not yet have been discovered. *Bridging in* moves us away from cognition into imagination, which is the realm of the archetypes, a term Jung used for innate patterns or designs that are universally

4   Kearney 1996, pp.54–55.
5   Edinger 1994.

inherited, and which inform our emotional experience. Each archetype has two essential extremes or opposites which are held together by a pull or a tension, balanced by the action of a symbol. These archetypes are encountered in Sesame through working with the embodied image. In practical terms, an archetypal tension is present when someone states, 'I had a great childhood and a wonderful mother who loved me dearly', only to discover that an opposite theme of destroying witch is repeatedly chosen in enactment. The split-off fear, pain and anger omitted in half telling the life story is released when the cruel or needy mother is discovered and given a space through a story. The shame that often denies a parenting wound is normalised and brought into a middle place, where it can find a way to be met rather than avoided.

The stories themselves are full of references to a journey between two archetypal places. In the story line of *Hansel and Gretel*, for example, the children are *bridged into* the deep forest by a conscious and very real famine in the land and the demands for nourishment motivating their starving stepmother. She leads them into a vast forest that is unfamiliar, where they have to encounter great terrors, darkness and imprisonment with the marauding witch in her confectionary cottage. To survive, Gretel has to outgrow a naive dependence on her brother and discover that she has her own strength and guile. Through her actions, both children escape but remain lost in the forest until they come to a lake, which has no bridge. The newly acquired qualities are trapped until a kindly duck spans the gap, carrying the children across the water to the other side. Once this transition is made, they know where they are and are able to find their own way home. They find the stepmother, once such a threat to them, unexplainably dead and her powerful reign over! It is now safe for them to forgive their father for his ineffective care, share riches and never go hungry again. In terms of a Sesame session, they have run the ritual of imaginatively entering a different archetypal reality, learning from it and returning with life skills that are tangible and effective. The inner forest journey has yielded resources with which to live in the outer world.

It is not only wounds of famine that can be met through negotiating the opposites: there is also the finding of latent abilities. If I arrive for therapy with a sense of low self-esteem and a loss of confidence for voicing my needs or opinions, a story such as *Mella* or *Jumping Mouse* may spontaneously draw me in. Taking a role in the story, I begin to share the archetypal pattern of a character's journey, a character who, like me, needs to break out of a restricting situation and go searching for a calling as yet outside my experience. In enactment, I have an opportunity to work towards owning a strength or quality which has not previously been recognised or affirmed. If I take on a character that represents the opposite to my habitual way of functioning, I make a start at constructing different meanings about myself, my relationships and my vocation. The intuitive choosing and subsequent embodying of a character or a story quality nudges me towards the next step to becoming more my whole self. Jung calls this the individuation process.

Bridges in a Sesame Myth and Fairytale session are, therefore, vital transition points, helping the archetypal opposites to come into balance. They span the gap between what is habitual and what is unknown, moving from the visible to the invisible, from the light into the dark, from the outside to the inside, from the surface to the depths. In these crossings, a relationship between the inside and the outside being encourages transformation and change. These bridges pass in and out of many archetypal lands. They are symbolised by some memorable images in literature – for example, the wardrobe leading into C.S. Lewis's Narnia[6] and J.K. Rowling's Platform 9¾ which opens the way to Hogwarts learning.[7] They are like Enid Blyton's Magic Faraway Tree, linking the earth to the ever-changing sky lands of magic. They enable a crossing to and from 'The Land' of Peter Slade. Stories hold endless metaphors for this place, which is as real and vital as the world of here and now.

Symbolic play with archetypes takes place in the *main event* or central section of a story enactment. Gradually, when moving physically through the story landscape and seeing with the eyes of imagination, a relationship with the invisible soul intelligence begins to awaken and people *drop down* into Kearney's *deep centre*, learning to trust this place in themselves. It is in the *bridge out* where reflection takes place, that the *as if* images of metaphor bring to mind word fragments, often having their origin much earlier in our lives. As we said, this deep work takes time and relies profoundly on *synchronicities* encountered after a session, sometimes days or months after, reinforcing and substantiating the process of learning that begins within the enactment experience. Jung uses the term *synchronicity* to indicate the way this new *information* projects itself on to outer circumstance, with the result that the outside self slowly makes conscious connections, 'gets it' and begins to change.

6   Lewis 1950.
7   Rowling 1997–2007.

Within the session, the therapist needs to be vigilant in guarding the space where the first nuances of the diffident soul story are expressed, through evocative word phrases and fragments of half-formed thought which have no erudite intellectual status, but which represent the harvest of psyche-logic. The second pillar of the bridge spanning the two psychic states has its foundations in the area of depth.

Creating bridges

The bridge in

In a Sesame session, the *bridge in* sits just before the *main event* and is designed to lead the group experientially towards what follows. The therapist has chosen the story from what she has observed of her client or group in the previous session, and in conjunction with the overall aim of the therapeutic work. If a movement session is planned as the *main event*, this *bridge* gives people a chance to experience a key motif of the movement quality or relationship that will be developed later. In a Myth or Fairytale session, the task of the *bridge in* is to prepare the way for the story, so that people are ready to hear the telling, having experienced something of the archetypal content before it begins. Through a short ritual or exercise using imagination, voice work, instruments, cloths or whatever the therapist feels to be appropriate, the *bridge in* prepares the way towards the core theme of the story, which will be encountered during the enactment that follows.

These are some of guiding questions that have to be considered when choosing *bridge-in* material. What is the therapeutic aim of the *main event*? How will the *bridge in* lead safely towards that? What specific energy or experience do I hope to offer people in the *bridge in* so that they are ready to participate in the story? Do I want the group to be in role for the story as they end the *bridge in*, or do I need to give them a mini-grounding so that they come back to themselves before listening to the story? An example may help here.

Working around the theme of autonomy with a group of Sesame students, early on in training, I used the African myth of *Kaang*. The story tells how the creatures are instructed by Kaang the Creator not to light fire. In the *bridge in*, an unlit candle and a box of matches were passed round the circle, with an instruction from me: 'On no account light the fire!' As can be imagined, there were all kinds of responses, but only once was the candle defiantly lit! Whatever the outcome, every student was in a relationship with the core motifs of autonomy:

conforming, separation and loss – all motifs that come into the story about to be told. The *bridge-in* experience brought these themes into the room and allowed the group to explore their individual feelings towards key motifs they were about to encounter in the story.

The other bridge, the *bridge-out* process, is much more complex.

Question: What do you understand by the term *bridge out* in a dramatherapy session?

> The way by which we tiptoe, stride, stomp our way, reluctant or willing, back to the present space and time

> Coming back from a place or state of being – a gathering of gems that one has collected from the visit and observing what use these have for you

> A magic call inviting people to cross back and then to recognise, realise, understand and accept conflicts in the mind

> Reflecting and speaking from one side to the other

> Linking from the imaginative creative place to the here and now

> A return from story or myth to my story

> A move to the place where we are accountable – a process of reflection, realisation and assimilation

> Between ordinary consciousness and other-than consciousness, walking out into the mundane, preserving the learning whether known or unknown

> Two perspectives – the insight for the client and the insight for the therapist

> Noting and letting what has happened be, living for days or weeks with the symbol that has come, as it repeats through my life.
> *(Response fragments from Sesame dramatherapists)*

The *bridge out* has two modes, the first being an *in-role bridge out* and the second a *de-roled bridge out*. They are determined by whether people are being asked to respond to the *main event* in character, or as themselves, having already stepped out of their roles. We will now look at the two modes.

The in-role bridge out

The story enactment part of the *main event* has ended and, if the enactment has been successful, it is inevitable that many emotions and energies, different for each person, will be in the room. People will sense a collective, group atmosphere, a quality that remains present at the end of the story, made up from a miasma of feelings, sensations, thoughts and hunches. The *in-role bridge out* works with this by setting up a form of embodied amplification, or a thinking in image, which is developed through the distance of the character, before de-roling.

The therapist works spontaneously here, tuning into whatever she perceives as being present. It is not her job to fix or sort things. To do so would be to meddle in a profound work that happens inside each person. The therapist's job is to allow time and space for personal responses, which have come to life through the enactment, to become ready to cross back over the bridge to the everyday. She has to be alert to notice the characters in front of her, their large and small gestures, intakes of breath, a turned-away anger, a stuckness, a fragile joy, tears or laughter. With a firm but sensitive manner, she enters the story world to dialogue with the participants, asking such questions as: Is there a part of the story that any character needs to re-enact? What does this character need in the re-enactment and how will this affect other story roles? Do any of the story beings have anything to say to each other, or do they have a question to ask? Is there unspoken love, rage, frustration which a character feels has been left unattended? Is there a wordless feeling that has been left neglected in one of the landscapes of the story? Will your character go towards or move away from that place? Did any character not have time to improvise a part of the story as they wanted to?

A re-enactment of the story, or part of it, can then be set up, followed by de-roling exercises and a grounding process, to draw the session to the end. There needs to plenty of time allowed for the *in-role bridge out*, as it often extends the enactment through giving characters the opportunity for further improvisation, still held within the container of the story structure. This mode requires flexibility and confidence in the depths process from the therapist, knowing her work is only to guide the group to a place where the process feels complete enough for the session to end safely. A few examples of the *in-role bridge out*, from the experience or clinical work of Sesame practitioners, now follow.

Example 1

The story

I was doing a parable called 'Sadness and Anger', in which the two characters swap clothes and are therefore hard to distinguish. One of my clients needed props to enact the undressing and re-dressing of the character and she grabbed some jumpers and coats. She ended up wearing her own coat when the exchange had been made, something that was not planned.

The in-role bridge out

The *bridge out* was about the removal of the coat, which was made more difficult as it was the client's own item. However, this was deeply meaningful and she talked about her inability to express her anger and the resulting depression, as symbolised by her wearing the coat in the group. The client realised that anger was underlying her depression (sadness cloaking her anger) and was able to embody aspects of anger, any sign of which she suppressed in her normal life.

Example 2

The story

In a one-to-one session with a child, over several weeks he explored defeating 'fear' or 'threat' in several different guises. I told a story about a fearsome giant and he engaged with killing the 'enemy', as he had before in many of his self-authored battles.

The in-role bridge out

During the *bridge out* we reflected on the ending. He moved to the sand play box, burying the giant partially in the sand and then swapping him for a smaller figure. The ending had changed, he told me. In his new form the giant did not appear so threatening and the villagers, no longer so afraid, invited him to join their community. Via metaphor, he seemed to be testing how it might be if this giant (as a symbol of fear) could be overcome in a different way, managed and lived with.

Example 3

The story

We were told the story of *Chiron the Wounded Healer*, and during the enactment I chose to embody him. I was overwhelmed with emotions and tears, but I kept on going, enjoying somehow the release of the psychic pain that I was carrying.

The in-role bridge out

During the *bridge out*, we created still images from the story and only then I clearly saw that I was being taught personally through the relationship I was making with archetypal content. The story allowed me to give a symbolic and poetic meaning to my psychic and physical wounds, and the connection with the archetype of the wounded healer gave me relief and confidence to move on with my studies by reinforcing my decision to become a dramatherapist, which I was questioning a lot.

The de-roled bridge out

The second *bridge out* mode is the one which happens after a de-role from character, when the return to the 'here and now' self has been facilitated. It is this bridge which is most used in Sesame work, simply because it takes less time.

Now the embodying of the story is over and the therapist makes a ritualised ending of some kind. It may be by holding a silence, or striking a singing bowl, or gathering what is in the room by describing it: 'So we are at the end of a story which has taken us into some powerful themes. In a moment, we need to find a way back to the room we all know, outside the story…'

The therapist is speaking directly to psyche, or, using the terms of archetypal psychologist James Hillman, to the soul.[8] She issues a warning that a shift from the imaginative state is now on the horizon. She is also addressing the ego when she says, 'There may be all kinds of responses that your character has had in playing their role. Don't worry too much about understanding this now. Simply find a way to notice

---

8   Hillman (1965, p.47) writes about how psyche and soul can be used interchangeably, suggesting that the term *psyche* is used more in relation to physical life, while *soul* on the other hand has metaphysical and romantic overtones. It shares frontiers with religion.

what wants to return with you from the story place…' At this point, the therapist stands on the bridge holding the landscapes of each territory and providing a *temenos* for soul and ego to be conscious of one another.

The *de-role*, like the session's final grounding which comes later, takes people back. It refocuses mind and body on the world of the five senses, returning attention to relationships with other group members in the tangible fabric of the room. A suggestion is then made by the therapist, asking people to reflect, perhaps to move, to sculpt, to draw or write their responses to the story enactment. There needs also to be a strong spoken reminder that this task is reflective and a clear remit about the non-performance nature of what is being asked. At this stage, just at the point of return from the spontaneous freedom of the imagined world, shame and the fear of judgment can slip in and close things down. The return to the conscious self, with its habitual demands and defensive positions, is being re-established. The familiar inner voices are beginning to make themselves heard. 'You know you can't draw.' Or 'I will make such a beautiful song out of this experience!' Or 'This reminds me of the anthropological paper I was reading last week where an argument was made for…'

The *doing* gets in the way of the *being* and tries to steal the potential for images to be perceived in the *bridge-out* time. The therapist needs to keep protecting and supporting the right of the inner to communicate either non-verbally or with a sketchy use of words. Each is an oblique option in the *de-roled bridge out* and neither is better than the other. The therapist can support a non-verbal process by suggesting:

> Think of the characters you have just played. Looking back at them, is there any insight they have for you for the rest of today? Show that through movement or a sound.

> Is there anything that you wish to leave behind from the story and anything that you would like to keep. Affirm this in a movement. This exercise is a Sesame (rather over-done) favourite!

> Take a moment in silence (or with a piece of music softly played) to reflect on the experience you have just had and what, if anything, needs to happen next.

To create a vehicle that will facilitate the process of bringing image back to words, she might say something like:

> Recall the story and select a moment which is still with you now… Use the crayons to remake that moment as a picture, nothing artistic,

just make it as it wants to be... If the picture had a name or a title, just for now and without thinking too much about it, what would that be? ... This name is a title for a two-line poem which can rhyme or not... If nothing comes – don't worry... Can you find a movement to express the poem which is ready to be shared with someone else? ... Share the movements and anything else that you would like to with one other... Bring anything that is left and wants to be talked about in the large group.

What image in the story caught your attention today? Sculpt that for yourself. Let this image write you a short letter with some good advice for you.

Are there any one-word responses that want to find voice as we come to end of the session?

This last process requires a period of at least ten minutes. The instructions will, of course, tune into what the therapist is observing and perceiving from the group. This style of *de-roled bridge out* allows people to make a first attempt to slowly bring words in. I will say more about the place of words and the wordless in Sesame work later. Here are some examples of the *in-role bridge out* from the experience and clinical work of Sesame practitioners.

Example 1

The story

I work with a man who has a poor memory, speaks with great hesitation and struggles to give news of his week. It takes a long time for him to find an idea or make a decision. Sometimes he will stand beside a chair waiting for someone to tell him it's OK to sit down. He had shown an interest in horses and had been visiting a stable, but for months he had been working up the courage to actually touch a horse. I introduced a story which involved a horse. He immediately asked to be the character who would ride the horse, and he rode it for a long time in the enactment.

The de-roled bridge out

I knew this was powerful because as we *bridged out* and reflected on the roles he had played, he showed no problem remembering the intricate details of what he had done in role or finding the words to describe his achievements. He kept bringing the idea of a horse into other stories, and eventually began riding a horse for real. His ability to remember enacting the role suggested it had been a big 'event' for him – more than his weekly news.

Example 2

The story

Working with a group of older people in the *main event*, the group told their own imagined creation story. Themes were of a religious and pastoral nature (brought by the group). Each client took turns to add a line or two of narrative and also to add something to the physical landscape. Following the creation of the land, they chose where they would place themselves within it and told stories which they believed would unfold in the land concerning travel, exploration and personal relationships.

The bridge out

The *bridge out* involved dismantling a landscape made out of textured materials (cloth, paper, cellophane, cardboard, etc.). During the dismantling of the 'river', a client spoke of things drying up and if the river is gone, then 'all life must be gone' – I was told that the remaining scene had to be dismantled quickly. Conversation within the group turned to nature, the seasons and death. This was the first time the group broached the subject of death directly and it seemed the imagined world gave rise to connections within their own stage of life.

Example 3

The story

Once in a story, I was a bridge which was crossed over by two tribes who lived on opposite sides of a chasm. They constantly sneaked across to steal treasure from each other. Every time, the bridge was broken down and then later rebuilt. Finally the bridge was left broken down.

The bridge out

I don't remember the *bridge out* because it did not work! I came out of the session feeling quite bruised and upset by being left in a broken state. Later I realised that my life as a housemistress, caring for 34 girls in an independent school, was exactly like a bridge between the girls and teachers, parents and house staff. The feeling I was left with was a sadness and of being broken down. Now, looking back, I see my creative spirit was being crushed by the daily pulling from the different groups. Recognising this helped me make a decision to take early retirement and retrain as a dramatherapist so my drama background could be used in a different way. This has led, eventually, to complete retirement and to working as a storyteller in the USA – a delightful way to live!

The last example above occurred during one of the Sesame Institute training schools. It illustrates a process which spilled from the *main event* into the *bridge out* and which left the session in an uncomfortable place. There was no language exchange during the school between me, as the trainer/therapist, and the student involved. We did not discuss or process it and, if we had, it is highly possible that the important discovery which she had to make would have been over quickly, tidied away into a rational soothing or making better. However, as she describes it now, the symbol of the bridge within the story of *The Bad People* and the quality it brought into consciousness were unfinished and raw. Situations must not always be resolved in the *bridge out*; Sesame work is therapy and feelings that come from an unsettled circumstance or event can mirror a specific life dynamic or struggle which births itself usefully from unconscious to consciousness, into awareness, the first step in making intentional changes.

Grounding

The experience of having shared a group and individual perception of a myth was very powerful. To be able to 'survive' my inner journey, to go through the vulnerability, to meet concealed elements of me and my past, and to come out accepting, embracing and connected to myself and my survival, is vitally validating. To share at the *de-role* the process of flicking off all those feelings, to discard them and place them in the centre – to see that other people are doing the same, and also holding those distasteful and painful experiences, gives me hope and strength. The therapist guides us and me – but it's my *own* hand I see, deftly throwing the residue of my experience to the centre of the circle. I am hearing it's OK to do this; actually that it is good to do this. I am aware of how much control I can now take if I wish to. I can do this discarding I am doing now, elsewhere – in my own way. This is a new possibility for me. The therapist leads us in faster exercises, and then she teaches us a song. I am back to my own body. My sense of powerlessness has been transformed. I am not passive anymore. I am vitally aware of my power and choice.[9]

The grounding

After the *bridge out* is completed, we are no longer in the land of the story. The *grounding* that follows has a very simple intention. It prepares people, physically and mentally, to leave the session. It does this by introducing practical exercises that employ the five senses and rational thinking. The therapist uses firm instructions and brings in concrete, left-brain learning tasks focusing on the body, the room and the other people around. As the writer above states, learning a song is a good way to collectively draw people's attention and voices back together.

Like the *de-role* discussed earlier, the function of the *grounding* is to leave imagined material behind, but there is a difference between the two forms. While the *de-role* can include use of creative art forms to draw out symbolic material, the grounding steers right away from the world of story and any hint of physical or imagined symbol. This part of the session is likely to take on different rhythm from what has gone before. Sometimes the therapist has to make a definite intervention to awaken an opposite or missing energy, which will facilitate people leaving the sessions safely. Obviously, the therapist needs to facilitate with sensitivity and not manipulate or tidy away the psychological affect of the *main event*, but her responsibility is to work directly, using practical exercises and ensuring that her manner and tone of voice attune to ending the group. If, for example, the *main event* has been ponderous and there is a heavy sense remaining in the room, she may need to work towards developing a contrasting lighter and faster tempo, through exercises that give this experience to the body. Knowing how to do this without taking from or denying what has gone before is a skill that grows

9   Quoted and used, with permission, from an email from a student participating in the Sesame Institute short course Introduction to Drama and Movement Therapy.

as the therapist comes to trust her ability to respond spontaneously, mindful that even when she gets it wrong, supervision can enable her to reframe the mistake. Consideration of such issues as transference and counter-transference can help her to use the experience as a relational starting point for the next session. The therapist's mistakes or failures in atunement often offer a chance for the client or therapist to talk mutually to each other, and these uncomfortable moments can become a time when the client is most empowered to speak honestly and become more collaborative in how the session is run.

Finally, the *grounding* does not involve imagination but the content of the exercises needs to be given creative attention. Repetition of a final ritual, perhaps the passing of a farewell gesture, or the extinguishing of a candle, are forms of recognised landmarks that people come to value when they are replicated week by week in the closing exercise. Within the Sesame community, there is a legacy of groundings handed from one generation to the next which are satisfactory because at some point someone creatively constructed them, specifically to end a session. Most people know the 'In, out, move on' circle dance, a simple and delightful movement piece created by the one-time course tutor Di Cooper, which appears and reappears over the years because it brings a sense of collective completion. Each therapist needs to do her own thinking on final rituals if they are to function well in engaging the five senses and not just be a habitual coda to what has gone before.

Chapter 4

Making Space for Soul Talk

Recent Research

Mary Smail

What is that you know

That you think

they don't know

and which you are afraid to tell them?

Esther Hicks Abraham[1]

The quotation above is from a YouTube video in which a therapist describes what she calls a new way of working with children on the autistic spectrum. She is excited about this work, but describes it diffidently, halting and stumbling as she talks about how her child clients have intuitively taught her to see, feel and know them, through what she calls 'vibrational interpretation'. She shyly proposes that this could herald a paradigm shift: that what the children have taught her is new and could bring fresh insight to what is already known about how people with autism relate to others. There have been significant breakthroughs in her therapy sessions, and parents are delighted with the changes they acknowledge are happening at home. The therapist is entirely convinced of the work but is disempowered when she thinks about how 'They' – her university faculty group – will receive her findings. She fears being judged as flakey, or being thought to be a 'woo-woo'.

The short clip goes on to show her consultation with a mentor who asks her the question, 'What is it that you know, that you think they don't know, and which you are afraid to tell them?'

---

1   www.youtube.com/watch?v=v4WAYJBDevw.

Bit by bit the woman answers the question, her confidence growing when she is supportively received, and she begins to talk more freely about her work. The mentor then gathers what has been said and repeats it back, using simple but coherent statements to describe the intuitive experience. Taken from a very different context to the one we are considering, the video is relevant to what I hope to convey here. It shows a previously silenced therapist, enabled by a process. Hearing her experience mirrored by another has accustomed her ears to what her previously edited-out voice is saying and helped her to find the respect that her discoveries deserve. She is now ready to go back to her contemporaries to share the originality of her research findings.

I use this little window because it mirrors something of the same challenge that faces dramatherapists as they deliver, describe and articulate their work in a world that says, 'Prove it!' David Read Johnson once wrote of the shame dynamics that can inhibit creative arts therapists as we strive to bring the creative forward in a concrete world of evaluation and consequent funding.[2]

Sesame therapists in particular, with almost half a century of obliquely and non-verbally using drama and movement in therapy, are at the 'softest' end of this. With our deference to the psyche, and a refusal to bow down too quickly to definition or explanation, our work is cut out! If we are to find a way to make a slow return to using words as part of the psyche-soul process, we need to get used to how soul thinks in patchwork fragments which can eventually be sewn together to make a garment, wearable in the world.

In Sesame, experiences of profound change, healing or insight have been somewhat cheesily described as 'golden moments'. If this makes you wince, please see it as a best attempt to describe the 'aha' reaction when an unexpected energy constellates through the story enactment or movement. 'Sesame Golden Moments' is a kind of hippy shorthand, a metaphoric word fragment to describe an effect that becomes actively present when something numinous breaks out, when something breaks through, comforts or confirms. While it is good that we have eyes to recognise this phenomenon, we need more words than 'SGM' to describe it in the world. We need language that enables us to stand by the transforming moment, without 'bigging it up', invoking some existing psychological theory or even inventing a theory of our own through the publication of grand papers! Publish or perish, someone

---

2   Johnson 1994, pp.173–178.

once said. Sometimes there needs to be a bit more perishing, or at best slowing down, before it can become possible to write authentically about the experience of psyche-soul. We need to feel towards humility in order to find the metaphoric language that returns us to the earth and ground of our being.

The challenge of finding words for what we do

As I write, I am aware of being at the task of finding vocabulary. I am attempting to articulate in a chapter what could be said just as well in one hundred words. The simplicity of what is being written about here is being 'bigged up' to contribute to what I hope is going to be a useful teaching book that will provide a resource for readers to explore their own way to dance and think with the ephemeral mysteries of the unconscious. But I task myself to find a way to stick by the simplicity of the active but wordless essence of Billy Lindkvist's founding dream, and the source at the heart of the SGM. I would like us to end with some thoughts on how we bridge image to words.

Reflective processing and half-formed articulation

> Logos when working beautifully leaves the soul out. If you bring the soul in, you start to stutter or you will go round in circles or you'll be unable to elocute it in a way that does justice to it – you will be in half darkness. My point is that soul means inferiority… Soul makes the ego feel uncomfortable, uncertain and lost. And that lostness is a sign of soul.
>
> *James Hillman, Inter Views[3]*

As I write, I am imagining my dear friend and mentor, Billy Lindkvist, reading about the place of talking in a Sesame session. Her impassioned cry rings in my ears: 'We do not interpret in Sesame! We are not psychotherapists!'

She is right, even for those of us who have trained and worked as psychotherapists while continuing to practise dramatherapy. And, looking back, I would say that my ability to make 'interpretations' was discovered less during psychotherapy training and more when learning to select material from what I interpreted from clients' participation, during training with Sesame!

---

3   Hillman 1983, p.93.

When teaching Myths, I remember a Sesame student asking at the end of a session, 'Is that it?' She had been left with things in the enactment that she wanted to talk about and was outraged that I had not set up an opportunity for dialogue. In this exchange she and I were both challenged. Hers was one of a series of voices that started me considering the place of talking in Sesame work. This question divides Sesame purists from those who make a plea for the importance of words to amplify and confirm embodied image and give it substance in the outside world. I believe this to be a necessary process for people of a more extraverted nature, people who process externally through hearing themselves talk, rather than introverting and containing. Sesame needs to address this question and make space for these preferences.

When teaching I began to ask the students to follow their one-hour experiential session in college with a brief time for people who wanted to speak about inner process. The timbre of this exchange was not about intellectual discussion. Students considered what conditions psyche-soul would need for a process I called *reflective processing* or *half-formed articulation*, a space for image to be spoken metaphorically through poetic word fragments, little lines of insight. They reflected on how to talk to one another from a liminal place, when an inner experience has not yet formed itself into rational understanding, yet can be amplified in the relational context of conversation.

Students slowly began to find the courage to learn how to set up safe conditions for *half-formed articulation* so that the outside, ego self would not steal the show by getting ashamed of the little fragments and 'big up' the psyche logic into knowledge. 'I have such a sense of lightness in my arm, I get the image of a great huge ship moving through me – it sounds so silly, I'm not sure why but I feel like a great blue light has been switched on' are examples of three metaphoric fragments that all were spoken after an enactment of *The Seal Woman*. It took courage for people to voice these, and courage was required for the therapist to trust that, whether what was said made sense or not, a patchwork of meaning was being created.

We found that if you assess this soul talk or inner thinking from a higher education perspective, you will find it unbearably messy and all over the place. It can either have an over-obvious, too-simple feel, or it can be strangely obscure and dream-like, appearing to make no connection with what has just been said. Soul-talk is deeply shy; there is a sense of *attempting* to form words and fumbling to communicate, which has a resonant emotional quality, but which keeps petering out. It feels embarrassing and uncomfortable: 'Sorry, this is complete rubbish' and 'I'm not making sense', often accompanied by a fanning of the face movement as a blush is cooled down. To people of a thinking type (*cf.* Jung's 'personality types') the experience of this phenomenon can be challenging because it is counter-logical, slow and apparently pointless. The depth pedagogy of the *half-formed articulation* is an emergent education which needs time and space for meaning-making to happen gradually. The word-grappling through talking or writing is the frontier at which psyche-soul turns symbol to metaphor, and metaphor to 'as if' words, ready to cross back over the bridge into the external world and be heard first by myself, then supported and shared with others. The therapist needs to have faith, trusting that through this process I have described meaning can emerge, changes are beginning to be felt and people's lives are being affected. Over and over again, she needs to set up a place for this kind of talk, affirming the non-intellectual poetic bias and nature of metaphoric conversation.

I asked Sesame practitioners to write about their use of *reflective processing* through *half-formed articulation*, both in their personal experience and in their clinical work. They each reported using the process, describing how they had understood it and made it their own. They named the fundamental requirement of a secure relationship between therapist and client, and the importance of intuitive attention to timing, before entering into the world of words. Nearly all agree that talking was an essential *bridge-out* option, but were hasty to balance this with reminders about the need for a wordless inner processing space, in a world that gives high praise to fast results and clarity. The following personal, or clinical, examples chart their work in practice with *reflective processing* in Myths sessions.

> Through reflective processing we begin to have a greater sense of what we have connected with in the story. Reflecting through embodiment or drawing, we can begin to process in a way that honours our feelings and emotions; we feel the image or the symbol emerging within our bodies, or we see it taking form on the paper. In this way firstly we experience the symbol/image from an emotional place and then begin to reflect on this experience in our thoughts, making a deeper emotional connection that is not reducible by deconstructive thinking. If words then emerge they, too, are from a non-thinking place and often they can take us by surprise. This

element of surprise provokes our reflective thinking on connections whilst maintaining a sense of depth.

I have found that the symbols which seemed important in the sessions were almost engraved in my body and stayed with me for days or months, autonomously and unexpectedly revealing their layers of meaning. At the same time, I have found that through looking at the material, sensing what has appeared intuitively, links are made between processes that might appear to be opposite. I have found that words or thoughts sometimes have as a starting point the pulse of the symbols, vibrating the essence of the session into the everyday life, translating images into action.

Reflective processing is about transforming an experience that you have had and thinking about it, how it may fit into your life and its process. By making a connection, this can allow a shift in behavior or at least some insight about one's own behavior, which can then be an ideal platform to effect change.

There is a need for sensitivity when choosing the right time to encourage and support the client connecting with the metaphorical across their life. If the therapist suggests this too early it could be intrusive and over-challenging. Once firm trust and continuity have been established, the client and therapist have the safety and greater confidence for reflective processing to take place.

I'm aware that I'm open and ready to 'make conscious' and time is built into the session for this to emerge if wanted. But I don't do it, believing what my teachers taught me, that the individual will know for themselves the how and when of illumination.

By guiding our attention, via the reflective means, the impression of an image or experience can evolve and entice new understanding. This process might occur in a revelatory moment or transpire over several days, weeks or years. Through writing, drawing, movement or silent reflection we hope to begin a kind of digestion where there is space for thought, linking the journey from image/s to word/s, which can then be transported with us and related outside of the session experience.

Colm Hefferon, an experienced trainer working in Dublin, attended a Sesame Introduction School in County Cork. He threads some of his half-formed reflective processing through writing after a session to describe his experience. It has been included here as first written and remains unedited:

> This work for me is a liminal space, indeed between the known and the unknown. It is a liminal feeling such as one sometimes experiences, but shies away from. In Sesame it is safe to do this sometimes. It seems to me that in both of the knowing and unknowing spaces, I was seeing my life not as me, but as my spirit guide which was inhabiting me at the time. Maybe it's a God space or Panoptic on space, which not only could I see as an observer, but in which I could also act as a participant. It had qualities of both. The observer came first. When it was safe the Doer was allowed in to change reality from a previous fixed to a present fluid. From cold to warm. From deadly to life-full.

Colm's writing comes from a training rather than a clinical context, but it emphasises how the therapist needs to hold back and allow the client time to process. If she does this, she is still working indirectly, symbolically and through the image, the key qualities of the Sesame approach, but letting the words in. Alyson Coleman speaks of Sesame practitioners as *highly trained companions* to the process of their clients. This aptly describes the relationship between therapist and client in a Sesame session and the safe place for soul fragments as a mysterious first fruit or hint of something new that is getting ready to incarnate.

After the session

So, to summarise, we are saying that we need to accustom ourselves to talking and thinking from an inner or psyche-soul perspective, and naming the cost of this because intuitive and emotional intelligence have not until recently been seen as valid ways of knowing. Happily, this is changing.

A recent documentary in which the nature of the self and the soul was being examined asked the question 'What is the soul?' The erudite scientist who responded to the question delivered his answer with contagious animation, but his words were half-formed. 'Well, it's not something we are taught. Its em…something inside us…em…a hidden thing. It's like innerness…an inner mental something…' An inner mental something! This final answer from the scientific academic was a fragment, a qualitatively fuzzy attempt to make sense of an unanswerable question. Through his body and his voice, however, he showed his response to the question. The answer was energetically or, we might even say, vibrationally present. There is something here that Sesame practitioners and the dramatherapy community as a whole need to consider as they explore different ways to show and demonstrate the efficacy of the dramatic arts as a healing therapy.

Stages of working with therapeutic myth enactment

I would like to offer two suggestions for how the therapist works with her counter-transference reflections on the story motifs and the half-formed fragments she has carried away with her to ponder after a session. Supervision, of course, plays an important role here and it is vital that the choice of supervisor enables the therapist to develop her knowledge of theory and outer world communication skills, as long as these are rooted in the source of healing, the psyche-soul. Here I would like to suggest a simple model offering six ways of looking at people who are working with story.

1. Initial assessment

Can the individual or group move into and use imagination, metaphor and embodied play? 'Try out' material is used to see if story resources will meet the needs of the clients or group.[4]

2. Embodied enactment

Can this person or group use projected play and take on a character or role? Is the client feeling comfortable enough to play and take on a small role or feature of the story? This is assessed by offering short story-making devices which are age-appropriate and short, rather than epic myths. This stage may need to be repeated, to see whether resistance or lack of confidence can develop, before the story work is extended. It can take time for people to actively choose or refuse a role, rather than adapting themselves to their ego defence patterns.

3. Role choices

Once a client is able to choose roles, the therapist can observe whether there is a pattern to the quality of the story roles chosen. Keeping

---

4   Smail 2004.

week-by-week notes on the parts people select, and symbols or qualities which emerge from the enactment, is a way of collecting fragments to see what texture or tone the patchwork is making.

4. Expanding role and spontaneity

Can the group/individual be autonomous in the enactment of characters, so that these are evolved through improvisation within the role chosen? What happens when a character is allowed to develop or flesh out their story environment or their character's motivation, while still holding the shape of the story? This provides a very useful means of exploring themes unlived in everyday life, but now obliquely being played out.

5. Story role reflection

Is there a mirror between the archetypal story role and personal experience? The therapist may notice that the client is choosing characters which directly link to his own story. By simply keeping this in mind rather than discussing it, a place in the conscious world exists for the client to come into his own relationship with a new insight or realisation.

6. Story role and life story changes

Is there an effect from the symbolic experience of the traditional story on the literal story of the person or group? At no time can the therapist push for this. However, there are times when someone may directly tell you how a story has touched something important in their life, or they may ask for more stories with a 'such and such' theme and in so doing intimate something that is alive for them psychologically.

The second suggestion is described aptly by Cath Butler as she writes about how inner thinking and theory can healthily marry in and be delivered to other health professions. She says:

> Apart from what emerges and begins to be processed in the session, how I do it is by noting internally and then in writing the symbols and metaphors that have come during a session, including all the physical and emotional manifestations of which I have been – or become – aware. Thinking, not necessarily verbally, may begin before literal recording. But as soon as possible, I write the notes. As I write, I am reflecting, and bringing words to the whole mind/body/spirit awareness that we seek to exercise in the session. A lot

of knowledge and experience can contribute to this, not only of symbol, but of the persons who have been involved in the session, including myself. The processing also, to me, takes place in the whole person, not just the verbalizing part. I can use movement, music and other art forms, as well as meditation, to aid the reflection, and to process what has been experienced. I believe that if the processing has been done, the whole, organismic self will take in hand what needs to happen next.

Clearly, there needs to be more work done in this area. Research is needed to find a way to let psyche-soul speak her backward healing imperatives, teaching obliquely by winding roads but with a fresh vibrancy that is transforming and compelling. We need to be careful that we do not fear research or see it as a job for other people in universities or laboratories. Everyone is able to re-search, to take a second or third look at their work and speak of it. We need to barge in on the research world, and participate in dialogue with existing researchers so that we can be confident and have a voice from which to describe our depth work. There are existing methodologies which I believe Sesame practitioners could use or revision to evaluate academically our way of working. The Sesame approach could safely be looked at through the lenses of client/therapist interviewing, journaling or the use of visual data. A phenomenological or auto-ethnographic methodology gives an acceptable academic name for processes that Sesame has been engaged in for years. Our quest must be to continue exploring existing research ideas and, if necessary, to create our own, so that we bridge the journey from inner to outer, and gird up our loins to speak rigorously of a therapy whose first voice is heard through the experience.

PART II

The Stories

in alphabetical order

ABU KASEM'S SLIPPERS

Iraq

Long ago in old Baghdad there lived an old miser called Abu Kasem. He was very rich but tried to hide this by wearing dirty old slippers. Everybody knew that he was a rich old miser.

One day he made a successful business deal. He purchased a quantity of crystal bottles for a song. Just a few days later he purchased a large supply of attar of roses. He celebrated by going to the baths.

An acquaintance tried to get him to purchase new slippers but he had no luck. After bathing, Abu Kasem went to the place where he had left his clothes. His slippers had disappeared and in their place was a pair, shiny, beautiful and apparently new. They belonged to a well-known wealthy judge who had arrived whilst Abu Kasem was in the baths. He wondered where the slippers had come from. Perhaps they were a present from a friend! Whatever the explanation, Abu Kasem drew them on. They would save him the trouble of shopping and bargaining for a new pair. With conscience clear, he left the baths.

When the judge returned, there was a huge scene. His slaves hunted high and low for his slippers but found only the tattered objects which everyone knew at once to be the disgusting footwear of Abu Kasem.

Abu Kasem was made to give back the judge's slippers. The court knew how rich he was and he had to pay a great deal to free himself from the clutches of the law. At least he got his own slippers back again.

Miserable and sorry, Abu Kasem arrived home and in a fit of temper threw his slippers out of the window. They fell into the Tigris, which crept muddily past his house. A few days later a group of fishermen thought they had caught a particularly heavy fish and hauled in their nets which had been ripped by the rough edges of the old slippers. Furious, they hurled the soggy objects through an open window. It happened to be Abu Kasem's. The slippers landed with a crash on the table where he had set out rows of crystal bottles filled with attar of roses ready for sale. The whole lot crashed to the floor and lay there, a dripping mass of broken glass and mud.

Abu Kasem cried out in great despair, 'Those wretched slippers! They shall do no further harm!' He took a shovel and went quickly into the garden and dug a hole in order to bury the slippers.

Now it so happened that Abu Kasem's neighbour was watching. He was always interested in what went on in the old man's house. 'He must have treasure buried there; otherwise his servants would be digging for him.' So the neighbour ran off to the Governor's palace and informed against Abu Kasem. Everything a treasure seeker finds belongs to the Caliph.

Abu Kasem was called before the Governor. His story of digging a hole to bury his slippers made everybody laugh uproariously. He was obviously guilty. In sentencing him, the Governor took the buried treasure into account and Abu Kasem was ordered to pay an enormous fine.

He was desperate. He cursed the wretched slippers. How was he to get rid of them? He decided to go out of town and drop them into a pond far away. As they sank into the water, Abu Kasem breathed a sigh of relief. But the pond was a reservoir which fed the town's water supply. The slippers swirled straight to the mouth of the pipe and blocked the water supply. Guards came to repair the pipe, found the slippers, recognised them as Abu Kasem's and reported him to the Governor. He was punished with a fine greater than the last. What could he do? He paid and got the slippers back.

He decided to burn them, but they were still wet. He put them on to the balcony to dry. A dog on the balcony next door became interested and jumped over and snatched a slipper. Whilst playing with it, he let it fall down to the street. It spun through the air and with considerable force landed on the head of a woman who was passing by. As it happened, she was pregnant. The shock and force of the blow brought on a miscarriage. Her husband ran to the judge and demanded damages from the old miser. Abu Kasem was almost out of his mind, but he was forced to pay.

Before he tottered home from the court, a broken man, he held the slippers solemnly aloft and cried, with a seriousness that all but reduced the judge to hysterics, 'My Lord, these slippers are the fateful cause of all my sufferings. These cursed things have reduced me to beggary. Please command that I shall never again he held responsible for the evils they will most certainly continue to bring upon my heart.'

AKINIDI AND THE COMING
OF HAPPINESS
Siberia

In the early days, when the world was young, Akinidi, daughter of the Sun, liked to fly around the heavens and look down on the creatures of the Earth, noticing that she could make them happy by shining her warmth down on them. She liked to watch the reindeer in the tundra, the birds of the air and the fishes of the sea becoming happy as they felt her warmth. But she noticed that people did not always react in this way. Some became happy when she shone her warmth on them, but others hid inside their tents and scowled. She became curious about people, wanting to find out why they were often unhappy and do something about it.

She went to her Father, the Sun, and said, 'I want to go down to the Earth. I want to find out more about people, why they are angry and sad. I want to make them happier.'

Her father tried to discourage her, pointing out that she was free to dance and sing in the spacious heavens, where she belonged. He warned her that people were difficult to understand, that they could be dangerous. But she would not give up her pleading and at last he gave in and said, 'Go to your bed and rest. You can visit the Earth tomorrow.'

Akinidi went to bed and slept. When she woke up, she found herself lying on a bed of animal skins, no longer a goddess but a young girl in the home of an old, childless couple. They were amazed to find her in their home. Akinidi told them she had come to stay with them and be their daughter and they were delighted.

They took her out and showed her round the island where they lived, in the middle of a seawater lake. The old man taught her to fish and to hunt. The old woman taught her to cook and spin, weave and sew. Akinidi was happy learning these things and her old parents loved to watch her as she danced and sang in the sunlight. When she asked if there were any young people for her to play with, the old man said, 'We are the only people on the island. You must stay here with us while you are a child. When you are big enough to wear the dress your mother is making for you, I will make you a crown of twigs and then you will be able to leave the island and meet other people.'

Akinidi realised she had been put on the island for her safety, while she learnt the ways of people. The old woman was making a dress for her out of plain, white fabric. Akinidi walked through the woods and along the beaches, gathering stones and berries of different colours. With them she created a beautiful pattern on the dress, astonishing the old couple, because in those days all clothes were made of plain fabric.

A day came when Akinidi was fully grown and her mother told her she could put on the dress. Her father made a crown of twigs and placed it on her head. He led her to the edge of the lake to see her reflection in the water. They could all see that she was beautiful. At that moment the island began to move, floating over the lake until it came close up against the land. Akinidi was able to step ashore. As she did so, her father pointed to a village in the distance, saying that when she got there she would meet a lot of people, some of them young like herself.

Akinidi embraced her old parents and walked away from them, towards the village. At the edge of the village she came to a big tent and stepped inside. A lot of people were sharing a feast. They were amazed to see the beautiful young woman in her many-coloured dress. Children ran to touch her. Women stroked her soft hair and the fabric of her dress. The men just watched, longing to embrace her. For a moment Akinidi reacted to the press of people like the goddess she was and turned into vapour so that people's hands passed through her. Then they all drew back, frightened. Quickly, she resumed her human form and reassured them, laughing as she led them out of the tent and down to the waterside.

There she gathered people round her and showed them how to sing and dance, something they had never done before that day. Then she invited them to sit by her and laid her hand on the ground in front of her, saying, 'What is under my hand?'

'Nothing!' they replied.

She lifted up her hand and they were amazed to see a pattern on the ground, like birds' feet, and two round circles, like the moon and the sun. They had never seen anything like it before. Very soon she had taught them to make patterns almost as good as hers.

This was how people first learnt to dance and sing and make patterns. Soon they were decorating their clothes with colours like

Akinidi's dress. Everyone wanted to learn these arts, so she travelled round the villages teaching them.

Wherever she went, she carried a little pouch of precious stones, bright and colourful, which she would sometimes give away. After a while, she began to notice some of the older people asking her for more and more coloured stones. She discovered that they were trading the stones for services, becoming powerful and idle. When Akinidi realised what was going on, she refused to give these greedy ones any more stones.

Then these old people began to turn against her. They were jealous of Akinidi and hated her for changing the old ways, teaching the young people to dance and sing and be happy. The angry old people went to find the witch Oadz, who lived in the swamp. They asked Oadz to help them get rid of Akinidi.

Oadz had been waiting for this moment. She also hated Akinidi because people no longer came to the swamp, asking for her advice and her spells. Many had turned away from her, preferring Akinidi's happy ways. Now she welcomed the angry muttering of the old people. She gave them a big moss stone and said, 'Go to Akinidi's tent and kill her with this stone. But be sure that you cover the smoke hole in the tent, so that her father, the Sun, cannot see what is happening. If he does, he will protect her!'

Seizing the stone, the elders hurried to Akinidi's tent where they found her playing with some children, teaching them a song. In their haste, they forgot to cover the smoke hole. They threw the stone at her chest, but she didn't fall. Instead, she turned into a vapour, hovering like fine grey smoke within the tent while one last song was heard, echoing round the walls of the tent and fading as the smoke drifted up into the sky above. In this way Akinidi returned to the heavens where she found her father, the Sun, waiting for her.

She was never seen on Earth again, but people went on feeling happy when they sang and danced and made beautiful, coloured patterns. Looking down on them from the heavens, the daughter of the Sun was happy with them, saying, 'You see, Father? Look what Akinidi has done!'

ALI BABA AND THE FORTY THIEVES
Medieval Arabic, Arabian Nights

Once there was a poor man who had lived well enough, but who had no access to a richness that had once belonged to him. The one resource that was always his was a certain tree in the forest which grew thick and green, not far away from the house where he lived. He would often walk to that place to repair himself and to rest alone where nothing would disturb him.

One day while he was in his tree-place, Ali Baba, for that was his name, heard the sound of riders. He saw a group of men dismounting from their horses and approaching a hidden rock face which he had never noticed before. One of them said, *Open Sesame*, and something opened to reveal a rocky entrance. Ali Baba watched each of the men pass through the door. The last one secured it with the words *Close Sesame*, and all was quiet again.

Ali Baba stayed hidden in his tree. After quite some time, he heard the muffled words *Open Sesame* on the far side of the door. The robbers came out laden, singing and cheering, with the richest gold and other things which sparkled and glowed. They mounted their horses and the captain shut the door saying, *Close Sesame*, and they rode away. When it was safe, Ali Baba came down and made his way to the rock face to try it for himself. *Open Sesame!*

It worked! Ali Baba entered a large cave, lit by light coming from a hole far above. He was surprised at this because he thought there would be only darkness inside and he fumbled at first, expecting to get lost. He made his way right to the back, and there it was. Treasure which I cannot describe, but which you would recognise because you know it well. Rich silks and deep carpets, silver goblets, great bags of money and, of course, gold. He gathered up all he could and made his way back to the door. *Open Sesame*, he said and the door opened. Ali Baba stepped out of the cave and made his way home, after closing the place.

The treasure he found was hard to keep. He did not know whether to hide it or show it. He was frightened about others if they knew how much he had. It took a long time for Ali Baba to work out just the right way to put the treasure to best use.

AMATERASU THE SUN GODDESS
Japan

A long time ago Izanami, the Mother of All, and Izanagi, the Father of All, gave birth to a beautiful little girl whose radiance filled the land with light. When her mother looked at her, she said, 'Our daughter is the most wonderful of all our children. We must not keep her here on Earth. Let us place her high in the heavens so that she may rule the sky.' And the young girl climbed high into the sky, to a place where she could look down on the lands below.

From that day she gave warmth and light to the plants and the animals. She taught the people how to weave cloth and how to grow rice and millet. The whole world loved her dearly. And they named her Amaterasu Omikami, which meant 'Great Shining Woman in Heaven'.

Amaterasu had a younger brother whose name was Susanowo, which meant 'Brave Strong Impetuous Man'. He ruled the mighty oceans. Susanowo wasn't like his sister. He was angry and loud and he stomped across the earth, tearing whole mountains up and making great valleys with his feet. His breath tore the branches off the trees.

One day their father called to Susanowo and said, 'My son, I gave you the seas to rule, but instead you tear across the land. You are too dangerous for the Earth. Since you cannot control your temper, I must ask you to leave.' Susanowo was furious. He stomped away from the land, straight up into Heaven.

Amaterasu greeted her brother, and when she heard about his exile from the world below, she invited him to live in Heaven with her. Susanowo promised his sister that he would behave better and thanked her deeply for her hospitality.

But it was not very long before Susanowo's behaviour reverted to normal and he was tearing up the land of Heaven just as he had done below. He chased his sister's precious horses, tore apart the rice fields of Heaven and smashed the irrigation ditches, ruining the season's harvest. He wrecked many buildings and smashed the beautiful mountains that Amaterasu loved to see from her home.

Finally, she could take it no more and fled. She ran to a large cave, ducked inside and pulled down a huge boulder to block the entrance. Suddenly, the sun was gone. Darkness closed over the lands of Heaven and Earth and everyone cried out, 'Amaterasu, come back!' But much as they cried and pleaded, the boulder never moved and Amaterasu never answered.

Then the gods and goddesses gathered outside the cave to discuss how they might persuade Amaterasu to come out. They came up with a plan and shared it with everyone. They gathered a lot of roosters outside the cave entrance and planted a large tree with hundreds of branches and they decorated it with bright cloth and banners. Then they made a ring of fire to drive away the darkness, climbed on top of an overturned barrel and danced a comical dance that set the crowd laughing.

Inside the cave, Amaterasu heard all these things going on. At last she called out, 'How is it that everyone is laughing when it is so dark outside?'

The gods and goddesses called back, 'Because out here there is a goddess who is as bright as you!'

Amaterasu became curious. She opened the door just a crack to see what was going on and looked straight into a big mirror that had been placed near the cave entrance. She saw that there was indeed another goddess who was just as bright as she. Amaterasu stared in wonder at her own dazzling reflection.

Then the gods gently took hold of her arm and drew her out to join the festivities. With Amaterasu out of the cave, daylight returned to the world. All the gods and goddesses cheered and the sky was blue again. The animals and the people were no longer cold. And soon the crops began to grow again.

The party went on and they all danced for many hours to celebrate Amaterasu's return. Susanowo was sent back to the ocean to resume the responsibilities he had been neglecting. And Amaterasu climbed back on to her throne, high in the sky. Once more the whole world gave thanks for her radiant beauty and bountiful gifts.

ASH

Native American

Once there was a man who had four sons, three of whom were his pride and joy and the fourth, Ash, who was squat, ugly and sleepy. He spent most of his time by the fire, gazing into the flames, just thinking. People called him names, but he didn't care.

One day, Whale-Man, the champion of a neighbouring village, issued a challenge to fight. Whale-Man was heavy with blubber and strong as thunder in a night sky. When he arrived, the village was covered in shame for there was no one willing to stand against him. Ash suddenly arose from the fire. The people thought he was crazy, but when they started to fight, Ash ducked through a hole in the wall and lured Whale-Man to follow. When he got stuck, Ash circled round, grabbed his feet and pitched Whale-Man, through the air, back to his own village. The villagers thanked Ash, but the brothers would have none of it and said it was a fluke. Ash said nothing, but there was a magic in Ash and magic does not like to be ignored.

Early one morning, a woman looking out saw that the trees of the nearby forest were lumbering towards the village, clawing up anything in their path. Panic struck as they came close and no one knew what to do. It looked as if the end had come. Ash did not stir from the fire, although he must have heard the screams. It was not until the trees were at his door that he raised himself drowsily and called, 'Stop that! Go back. You can trust me. There is no harm here.' The trees faltered and came to a halt, and then they picked up their roots, turned round and made their way back to their own ground. People applauded Ash, but the brothers would have none of it, and the magic in Ash noticed their denial, for magic does not like to ignored.

Not so very long after this, the weather changed and the air was filled with sound. The mountains were collapsing and toppling haphazardly down into the village, rock by rock, destroying homes and creatures alike. This time the villagers shouted for Ash, but he lazed by the fire, as if not hearing. They went to him and made him wake up. Ash called to the mountains, 'Stop that! Go back. You can trust me. There is no harm here.' And the mountains stopped immediately and built themselves up and returned to their source. Ash was truly celebrated. 'If only we had his wisdom. If only we had this magic in us,' they said. But the brothers looked away, and the magic in Ash did not like being ignored.

Two moons later, strangers arrived to the village. They were not hunters, nor had they come to trade beads. They would speak to no one but went straight to the hut of Ash and told him that the Master was waiting. Ash raised himself immediately and walked with the strangers, who took him away in their boat. No one understood what this meant, except Ash's father, who wept bitterly.

The strangers took Ash to a cave beneath the setting sun, down through to the sea bed. There lay the Master, a man so old that his body was all but gone, though his eyes were alive and bright. It seemed that he was pinned to the ocean floor, for a huge pole pressed down on his chest and soared high above, quite out of view. When he saw Ash, he said, 'You've come at last! I have held everything in place for a thousand years and no one has come to help. But you have enough magic in your soul which makes you ready.' And Ash lay down beside the old man and gladly took the pole and held it firmly. For the magic in Ash was recognised and had found its place.

THE BAD PEOPLE

Sesame Original

Long ago and far away there was a village.

The people of the village kept a precious sack of gold and other treasures deep underground. Sometimes they would take something out of the sack and have a feast. There was always plenty left. Nobody knew all that was in the sack.

One day all the men of the village went out hunting. When they got back, the treasure was missing. The old grandmother had seen the theft. She told them that the treasure had been stolen by the Bad People who lived on the other side of the valley. To get it back, the people of the village would have to follow the Bad People through the woods and cross the river and a big field of deep grasses, to the cave where they kept their precious belongings.

The hunters decided to go straight away and get the treasure back. They travelled a long distance through the woods, and when they reached the river, they had to build a bridge over it before they could get across. On the other side they met an old person and asked him if he knew the way to the Bad People's cave. The old person pointed to the field with the deep, thick grasses and said the cave was on the other side of that field. But they would have to be careful because it was always guarded. The guard on duty always marched up and down in front of the cave, looking out for anyone who might be approaching. However, when he had crossed the mouth of the cave, he always stopped for four seconds before turning round and marching back again. The only way they could get into the cave was to wait for the moment when the guard's back was turned and make good use of that time, first to creep through the grass until they were close to the cave and then to slip past him, one by one, when his back was turned.

Once they were inside the cave, they would have time to look around, and when they had found the treasure, they would again have to get past the guard with the sack, taking advantage of those four seconds when his back was turned. They would have to dive back into the long grass and carefully make their way through it to safety, always making sure that they only moved when the guard had his back to them, all the way to the river. They must not stand up and run until they were safely on the other side of the bridge.

The hunters thanked the old person and did exactly as he told them. They made their way stealthily through the long, deep grasses, creeping along on their stomachs. They found the guard marching up and down, and they slipped into the cave behind his back, one by one. And there was the treasure, in a sack, for them to take with them out of the cave and safely away, through the long grasses and home.

When they got back with the sack of treasure, they celebrated its return with a feast. Then they put it in a safer place and made sure that it was never stolen again.

BEAUTY AND THE BEAST

French Fairytale, Perrault

There once was a merchant with three daughters, one who was vain, one who was spoiled and a younger one whose name was Beauty. The merchant's business had fallen on hard times and he had to go to the city. He asked what each girl would like brought back as a gift. The vain daughter asked for a mirror which would reflect and extol her as the most beautiful woman in the world, while the spoiled girl asked for a ring which would exemplify her richness. But Beauty, when pushed, asked for only a single rose.

The merchant's city business failed so there was no money to purchase gifts. A storm broke out on his journey home and, losing his way, he allowed his horse to choose the path. They ended up at the front door of a great and ancient palace. The merchant called, but no one answered. He cautiously entered and found a sumptuous meal was waiting for him, and in an upstairs room a cosy bed had been warmed and prepared.

The next morning the merchant saw a rose bush. Remembering Beauty, he picked a rose, but as soon as he had done this, a wild creature, grotesque and beastlike, began to attack him, accusing him of treachery and theft against hospitality. When the merchant begged to explain about Beauty, it was agreed that he would be saved, on the condition that he send her to the palace to live with the Beast. On the merchant's return home, Beauty gladly received her rose, but when she heard what her father had done, she knew his promise must be honoured and her fate was set.

Everything Beauty wanted was in the palace, but she never met a soul and she became deeply lonely. One day when she was in the library, writing appeared on a mirror. She wrote back. Each day she conversed with the mirror writer. Later on she heard a voice in the garden which spoke to her. She told the voice, 'I would so like to see you', but he refused her, saying his appearance would harm. Beauty begged the voice to show himself, but when he trusted her and first appeared, she fainted away with horror. The Beast was wounded to the core, but in time Beauty began to love him as he was. It was when he asked her to marry him that she did not know what to do next.

Beauty wanted time to visit her father's house again. The Beast reluctantly agreed, on condition that she would return to him within a week. If she failed, he would die. Beauty agreed and returned home with wonderful gifts for her family. Her sisters were jealous of her beautiful clothes, her riches and her joy. So they turned the house clocks back by two weeks so that Beauty would unwittingly break her promise to the Beast. But he called to Beauty in a dream and she remembered and immediately made her way back to his palace. She found him by the rose bush, all but dead. She held his poor body close to her own, telling him of her love for him. A tear from her eyes fell on him as she spoke his name. Very slowly, the body of the Beast softened. His creature skin fell away and he took the form of a fine young man. The love of Beauty had broken an old spell, and from then on he and Beauty lived happily together, ever after.

As for the sisters, it is said that they became statues and remained that way until the day when they could own and remember their own faults.

THE BOY WHO LIVED WITH BEARS

Native American

There was once a boy whose mother and father died, leaving him in the care of an uncle. His uncle was a huntsman who had no time for children. He left the boy alone all day and ignored him in the evenings, feeding him scraps and making him sit in a cold corner away from the fire. But the boy never complained, as he had been taught to respect his elders.

Even so, the uncle felt that he was a nuisance and made up his mind to get rid of him. He said, 'You can come hunting with me today.' The boy was pleased. The uncle led the boy deep into the forest until they came to a cave. The cave opening was small. The uncle told the boy to crawl inside and drive out any animals that were there. The boy crawled into the cave but found no animals. Then he saw his uncle pushing a big stone across the cave entrance. He called out but no one answered, and he realised that his uncle had left him trapped in the cave.

At first he panicked but he remembered his mother had once said, 'If you are strong and have faith, good things will come to you.' Remembering this made him happy and he sang a song to keep up his courage.

After a while he heard sounds of scratching and squeaking near the cave entrance. Listening hard, he could make out voices saying, 'There's someone inside. It sounds like he needs our help.'

The stone was rolled away and light streamed into the cave. He crawled towards it and found himself safely outside, surrounded by animals. A small voice said, 'Now we have rescued you, we are going to look after you. You must choose which of us you would like as your family.'

The small animal that had spoken was a mole. There was a huge elk. There were deer and squirrels and rabbits and lots of other animals, standing in a circle around him. The boy said he didn't know how to choose. So the animals told him something about themselves to help him decide.

The mole said, 'I live under the earth. It's dark and cosy and we have plenty of worms and grubs to eat. Come and live with us!'

The boy replied politely that he was too big to enter the mole's tunnels and he didn't think he could live on worms.

The beaver spoke of the joy of living in water and eating the bark of trees. The boy didn't think he could manage that either.

Nor did he think he could he keep up with the deer as they ran through the forest, feeding on grass and twigs.

Then the old mother bear said, 'We bears move slowly, and though our voices can be harsh, our hearts are warm. We eat berries and roots. In winter we curl up together and sleep. If you come with us, our fur will keep you warm.'

The boy felt he would like to be a bear. He joined the bear-woman's family of bears and, from playing with the bear-woman's two cubs, he was soon as strong as a bear. He lived with them a long time.

One day when they were out looking for berries, the old bear-woman told them to be quiet and listen. They heard a twig snap and she said, 'He is the heavy-footed hunter. The twigs and leaves tell us when he is coming. We have nothing to fear from him.' Another time they heard a man singing and she said, 'That one doesn't know that everything in the forest has ears. He could never catch us.'

But a day came when the old bear-woman said, 'Listen! This one is dangerous. He has a dog and never gives up until he has caught the animal he is after.' Then they heard barking and the bear-woman said, 'Run for your lives! The four legs has caught our scent.'

They ran and ran until they were exhausted. Then they hid inside a hollow log. When the dog came sniffing at the end of their log, the bear-woman growled and the dog drew back. The boy smelled smoke and knew that the hunter had made a fire to smoke them out of their hiding place. He called out loudly, 'Stop! Do not harm my friends!'

The man shouted back, 'Who is that speaking? Is someone human inside this log?'

The boy crawled out and recognised the hunter as his uncle. The man was amazed. He told the boy how he had gone back to the cave that day, regretting the terrible thing he had done and, finding no one there, believed that he had been killed by wild animals. He was overjoyed to find his nephew safe.

Then the boy told him how kind the animals were and how the bears had looked after him. He said, 'They are my family now. So you mustn't harm them.'

His uncle promised to be a friend to bears from that day on. The bears were still frightened, but the boy reassured them and they came out of the log. Talking to the boy, in words that sounded like growls, the mother bear said it was right for him to return to his own kind, now that his uncle wanted to look after him. She told him that the bears would always be his friends and that he must never forget the warmth of an animal's heart.

The boy went back to live with his uncle, but they had to find a way of life that didn't depend on hunting. And the boy remained a friend to animals for the rest of his life.

CAP-O'-RUSHES

English Fairytale

A rich man had three daughters and he asked each one how much they loved him. The first said as much as life; the second, as much as the world; the third, as much as meat needs salt. The man was outraged by this last reply, thinking his third daughter did not love him and was being rude. He sent her away.

Outcast, the girl made herself a hat of rushes, to wear over her fine clothing so that she would not be known. She wandered until she came to a castle where she begged a job in the kitchen, and they called her 'Cap-o'-Rushes' because she would not tell them her real name.

One day, the servants went to watch the rich people who were attending a ball within the castle. Cap-o'-Rushes said she was too tired to go, but when they were gone, she took off her rushes and made her way there. The master's son fell in love with her, but she slipped off and could not be found. On two more nights this same thing happened, but on the third night he gave her a ring and said he loved her and he would die without her.

As there were no more balls, the master's son took to his bed because he had lost his love. Orders were sent to the cook to make some thin soup to nourish him, and Cap-o'-Rushes pleaded to be allowed to make this. When permission was granted, she popped the ring he had given into the soup and he, of course, found it as he drank. He demanded to know who had cooked the soup, and Cap-o'-Rushes was summoned. He questioned her until she told him that she was the lady at the ball and he recognised her when again she removed her rushes.

Before long they were wed, and Cap-o'-Rushes insisted that the wedding feast be prepared without any salt. This meant that all the food was without flavour, and her father, who was a guest, suddenly realised what his daughter had meant. He burst into tears, now fearing she was dead. Cap-o'-Rushes told him that she was his daughter, and so they lived happily ever after.

CHIRON THE WOUNDED HEALER
Greek Myth

Chiron was born after his father Cronos, an immortal God, took on the form of a horse so that he could seduce Philyra, a pretty mortal woman. He did this so that his wife would not recognise the adultery and see what was going on! Chiron was born then as a centaur, half man and half horse, half mortal and half divine.

When Philyra birthed Chiron, she abandoned her child, rejecting him on sight and leaving him motherless and quite alone. Eventually, the great God Apollo took pity on the infant and nurtured him, teaching him how to create poetry, the rules of sports, how to sing and play the lyre, how to think and create good order, and how to fight. Eventually, Chiron became a skilled teacher. Jason, Hercules, Asclepius and Orpheus were just a few of the great heroes of the land who came to him to be taught, when they were young.

One day, there was a wedding celebration which went on for days and nights, and the centaurs, with whom Chiron lived, became drunk. A fight broke out and, intending to calm the brawl, Hercules fired a poisoned arrow into their midst. To his horror, it hit Chiron, piercing him deeply in his leg. From that day on, whatever Chiron did, the wound of the poisoned arrow would not heal, and because of his immortality he was unable to die from the pain he suffered. He spent his days searching among the fields and forests for herbs that would comfort or heal him. The poor and the sick, those in pain, came to visit him and received consolation from his wisdom. He became known as the wounded healer who could give healing but was unable to heal himself. This went on for years.

Hercules was consumed with guilt and sorrow about what had happened to Chiron. He decided that he would go to Zeus, King of the Gods, to appeal for help. Plead as Hercules would, there was nothing that Zeus could do except to suggest that if Chiron were willing, he could surrender his immortality, by descending to the underworld and releasing Prometheus, who was tortured by a creature who tore out his liver by day, only to have it grow back again by night. This was his punishment for once cheating the Gods and stealing their fire. However, if Chiron would embrace the underworld and so lose the pain of his wound, Prometheus could go free. Chiron agreed to this.

Making his way to the mouth of the underworld, Chiron descended by way of the river Styx, and was ferried across the shady water by Chaeron the boatman. He was taken down and down to the most desolate corner of that land, a place named Tartarus, where he stopped. There, without what had ever been known to him, without any hope of what might be, reabandoned into a place where even death shades and whispers slowly skulked away from him, he was disposed into the annulling silence of infinite night. He stopped with nothing, in the voiding numbness of that place, without breath, without feeling and without pain.

After nine days, Zeus recognised the suffering and sacrifices of Chiron and took pity. He raised Chiron to the heavens and placed him in the sky as a constellation of stars called Centauras. We now know him there as Sagittarius or as the little-attended planetoid Chiron, placed within the outer solar system of planets and suns to guide us into healing.

COYOTE AND THE LAND OF THE DEAD
Native American

Early in the life of the world, Coyote visits Eagle. Eagle's feathers are rumpled, the cooking pot is empty, the fire has gone out. He is sad. His wife is dead.

Coyote sits with Eagle and thinks about death. Why does everyone have to die? He decides that he and Eagle will journey to the land of the dead and bring back Eagle's wife. Eagle says, 'Let's go now.'

They set off to the west, over the mountains. At night they listen to the spirits of the newly dead. At length they come to a grey flat land divided by a river. Beyond the river is the land of the dead. They see a village.

Coyote shouts for a boat. Eagle joins in, but there is no sound. Coyote begins to sing, a song he feels he has always known. Four men come with a canoe in rhythm of the song. Coyote and Eagle step into the canoe. The canoe moves silently through the mist. Eagle questions them – but the men are silent.

Eagle and Coyote step out. The moon rises, casting a pale light. On the edge of the village, dark, silent figures await them. An old woman steps forward. She tells them they are in a sacred place – a place not for the eyes of the living. She guides them to a lodge made of thick mats, where a small fire is burning. When they go inside, the doorway vanishes; there is no way in or out. 'Are we prisoners of the dead?' Eagle asks.

They begin to claw the walls, but it is no use. The walls can only be broken with an implement of the land of the dead. Suddenly, food is brought. Eagle and Coyote gulp the food. It is chicken, and Coyote keeps the last bone in his mouth.

'When are we to be allowed out of this lodge?' Coyote asks. There is no answer. With the bone, Coyote begins scraping the mat to make a hole. Finally, they peer through. From the centre of blackness they hear a powerful song. It brings back memories for Eagle and Coyote.

The moon begins to swell. Every part of the village can be seen more clearly than day. When the moon's light is brightest, the dead begin to gather, finely dressed. They join in the song. Eagle sees his wife.

Coyote goes over to a pile of antelope hides. Eagle watches his wife. Coyote takes a splinter of bone and one of his hairs and sews the antelope skin to make a bag. Then he peers through the hole.

Coyote begins to sing a song. He smothers the singing of the dead. The moon shrinks. Coyote stops singing. The dead become very motionless. Coyote enlarges the hole and they slip through, dragging the bag with them.

Coyote lifts the spirits of the dead and puts them in the bag. The sack remains light. He brings the spirit of Eagle's wife last. Eagle is anxious. They must be back before dawn.

At last they reach the river. Coyote finds the canoe. The sky is growing lighter. They step into the canoe and begin to move towards the shore. Eagle says, 'What will happen when the dawn comes?' 'The dead will awaken and they will have weight,' Coyote replies. The sky is lighter. The far shore looms up. The dead begin to awaken. The bag moves and sways. The canoe tosses and turns. All their voices rise in an outcry, and all tumble into the river. Coyote turns the boat towards the shore. They reach the shallows and stumble on to the land of the living. The dead become untangled. All stand before Coyote and Eagle.

Coyote says, 'We have brought you back to the land of the living. You may return to your homes.'

The dead smile quietly. The old woman says, 'We understand your intentions, but we have no wish to return. We love the peace and stillness. This helps us to gain wisdom which leads to understanding.' The dead move to the canoe, the wife of Eagle last.

'Do not grieve for me,' she says. 'Some day you will stay with me for ever in the land of the dead.'

Coyote and Eagle stand on the shore and watch the spirits of the dead move across the river to their chosen land.

CREATION MYTH OF THE MAYANS
Guatemala

At first there was chaos. Great mists everywhere. Then the chaos separated into three parts: the sky, the earth and the underworld. There emerged the ancient spirits – the gods.

The gods gathered to discuss their plans for creating life on earth. First, they created plants, mountain spirits and animals. The gods considered their work and were pleased. 'Now there is life on earth!' they said. They commanded the plants, mountain spirits and animals to praise the gods who had created them.

But the plants and mountain spirits had no voice. Only the animals could make sound. They cackled, mooed, barked and neighed; they grunted, roared, hissed and bellowed, each animal using its own voice.

The gods were displeased; no animal could pronounce the names of the gods who had made them. Again they gathered in council and decided to create men and women in their own likeness.

It was difficult. First, they made men and women from wet mud – when the rains came, the mud people were broken up and washed away.

Then the gods carved men and women from wood. They made wood puppets who were able to move and walk, but they had no powers to feel and think – no knowledge of their creators. And the gods were displeased and sent a mighty flood and drowned the puppet people they had made.

When at last the flood waters subsided, three pairs of twins emerged from the mud. Each had magical powers. But they were cruel and evil; they refused to praise the gods. They plotted to defy the creators of life.

The gods were angry. They sent thunderbolts from the sky to strike down and destroy the twins that had arisen from the flood.

For a long time after that, the gods abandoned the earth. They forgot the plants, the mountain spirits and animals that still inhabited it. At length the gods decided on a last attempt. They gathered again in council. After a long discussion they decided to appeal to the animals for assistance, for the animals had flourished and were wise.

The animals were pleased when the gods consulted them. They led the gods to a magical plant that grew in a secret place. With the aid of the plant, the gods were able to create men and women. They gladly praised the gods. At last the ancient gods were content.

DEMETER AND PERSEPHONE
Ancient Greek Myth

Demeter, goddess of the harvest and all growing things, had a daughter called Persephone who always helped with her work, tending the fields and the orchards. Day in, day out, the two goddesses went about their work together.

One morning, when Demeter was getting ready to go out and work in the fields, Persephone said, 'I don't want to go to the fields with you today. I want to visit with my sisters, the wood nymphs, and play among the trees and the wild flowers in the meadow.'

Demeter was sad at the thought of a day without her daughter, but she wished her a happy day and went off to the fields on her own. Persephone ran to find her sisters and all day they danced and played together among the trees. Towards evening, Persephone found herself at the edge of the wood, looking at a meadow studded with wild flowers. It was so beautiful that she forgot about the game she was playing and wandered out among the flowers, entranced by their colours and shapes. There was a deep purple flower with a nodding head that she could not resist. She reached out to pick the flower and the earth at her feet cracked open. There was a rumble like thunder coming from under the ground, getting louder and louder. A chariot drawn by black horses and driven by a fierce charioteer burst out of the ground and Hades, the King of the Underworld, looked down from his chariot, entranced by her beauty. At once he recognised that Persephone was the one he needed to be Queen of his dark kingdom. He leant over and swept Persephone off the ground, placing her beside him in the chariot. Though she begged him to let her go, he held on to her and drove on at great speed.

They raced across fields until they came to the side of a river and Hades had to rein in his horses. Persephone thought she might escape at this point, but Hades threw a thunderbolt at the river and a huge chasm opened up in front of them. He cracked his whip and the horses plunged in, galloping down a dark tunnel into the Underworld. The waters of the river water closed over their heads and not a trace of them was left.

As evening descended on the Earth and there was no sign of Persephone, Demeter went out to meet her. She asked the wood nymphs where Persephone was. They said they had lost sight of her when she wandered into the field of wild flowers. Demeter walked into the meadow but there was no sign of her daughter. Then she knew that something mysterious had happened and she would have to look for Persephone. She went home and disguised herself as an old woman, leaving her work in the fields to set off on her quest.

In this disguise, Demeter travelled through Sicily and Italy and came to a well by the road, just outside the city of Athens. Here she stopped to rest and watched as three young women came to draw water. They talked with her and, discovering that she was on her own, asked her to come home with them and help with their baby brother, who was sick. In return they offered her food and shelter. Demeter agreed to go home with them and help with the baby. As soon as she began nursing him, the colour returned to his cheeks and he was soon fat and well. Demeter had become fond of the baby boy and, being a goddess, she conceived a plan to give him immortal life. One day when she was alone with him, she started to perform the fire ritual. As she came to a point in the ritual when the naked child was laid in the fire, which would make him immortal, his mother came into the room, saw what she was doing and snatched the baby from her arms. Demeter threw off her old woman's disguise in a rage and said, 'You stupid woman! Your son would have been immortal if I had completed the ritual. Now he will die a mortal death like everyone else!' She swept out of the house and continued on with her journey.

Leaving the city of Athens behind her, Demeter walked out into the country, asking people as she went if they had seen or heard anything of Persephone. At last she came to the river bank where Hades had thrown his thunderbolt. She walked beside the river, making her way upstream, and came to a little spring that gurgled and sang in the sunlight. She stopped to listen and the spring said, 'Dear goddess Demeter, I have something to tell you, something no mother would wish to hear. Persephone is a prisoner of Hades, King of the Underworld. He found her among the wildflowers and carried her away to his kingdom.'

Demeter was filled with anger. She went straight to Zeus, most powerful of the gods, and said, 'Oh Father Zeus, do something to help me. Persephone, my daughter, is a prisoner of Hades. He has carried her away to the Underworld. You cannot allow this. Make him return her to the Earth where she belongs.'

Zeus did not want to intervene. Hades was as powerful in the dark Underworld as Zeus himself in the world above, and together they held the powers of light and dark in a delicate balance that he didn't want to disturb. But Demeter wouldn't give up. She threatened that if Persephone did not return to her, she, Demeter, the goddess of all growing things, would neglect her duties and there would be no food. Everyone in the world would starve. When he heard this, Zeus recognised that in her grief Demeter could do great harm to his kingdom, the Earth. So he relented, saying, 'This much I can do for you. If you go down to the Underworld and find that Persephone has not eaten since she went down there, she can return with you to the Earth. But if any food has passed her lips since entering the Underworld, she will have to remain there.'

Demeter set off for the Underworld immediately, descending into the dark earth until she came before the throne room of Hades. She found him seated on his throne with her daughter, Persephone, seated beside him. Persephone rose to embrace her mother. Demeter returned her embrace and then she drew back, saying, 'Persephone, my daughter, have you eaten anything since you came into this dark place?'

Persephone did not reply, but Hades said, 'This very morning your daughter ate six pomegranate seeds. It is the first food she has eaten since coming into to my kingdom.'

Demeter left without another word, going straight back to Zeus to declare that she would not accept the loss of her daughter for six pomegranate seeds. She said, 'If you do not let her return to me, I will not attend to my work. Nothing will grow on the Earth again, no fruit, no cereal crops, no flowers. I cannot tend the earth without Persephone. I am too sad to bear fruit.'

Great Zeus heard the grief in her voice and knew that she was speaking the truth. He recognised that, without Persephone at her side, Demeter would lose heart and be unable to tend the Earth. And so, for once, the all-powerful god tempered his judgment. He decreed that because Persephone had eaten six pomegranate seeds she must spend six months of the year in the Underworld, but at the end of that time she could return to the Earth and tend fields and orchards with her mother.

So it came about that the Earth experiences winter as a grey and barren time when Demeter grieves over her daughter's absence, but as winter draws to an end Persephone returns, bringing with her the joys of spring, and her mother greets her with sunshine and with flowers. The birds sing of happiness and the Earth produces its fruit and harvest. But this happy summer time is inevitably followed by autumn. The days grow shorter and colder and Persephone says goodbye to her mother, returning to spend the six months of winter with Hades, her husband in the Underworld.

ELIDORE
Wales

A boy called Elidore lived at St David's, on the west coast of Wales, where he was being educated to be a monk. He lived a little way from the monastery with his widowed mother and every day he would trudge up to the monastery school. Every day the monks struggled to teach him his letters and numbers, but Elidore found learning difficult. His attention often wandered and then the monks would beat him, but the more he was beaten, the less he seemed to learn.

One day, when he was twelve years old, Elidore was on his way to school and suddenly he couldn't stand it. He turned off the path and walked into the great forest near St David's. There he wandered about for a day and a night and another day, eating nothing but nuts and berries. Towards evening on the second day, he found himself on a riverbank with a cliff behind him and, in the side of the cliff, a deep, dark cave. By now he was so exhausted that he just lay down and went to sleep. He was woken up by the sound of voices and saw two little men talking near the entrance to the cave. When they noticed that he was awake, they came over and asked who he was and what he was doing there.

He told them his name was Elidore and that he was supposed to be at school with the monks, but he couldn't face it any more because he found learning too difficult and didn't like being beaten when he got things wrong. The little men said, 'Then you must come with us. We come from a country where everyone plays games and sports and nobody goes to school.'

Elidore followed them through the cave and down a long, dark tunnel. At last they came out into a beautiful country with hills and rivers, woods and trees. It was very different from the country he knew, green and lush but overcast, with never a break in the clouds to see the sun by day or the stars by night. All the people were small, not dwarfs but perfectly proportioned with fair hair down to their shoulders, many of them riding small horses no bigger than greyhounds.

The little men announced that they were going to take Elidore to meet the king. They led him to the king's palace, up a staircase and into a beautiful throne room. The king was seated on a throne and was as small as they were. He welcomed Elidore and introduced him to his son who was, he said, in need of a companion to play with. The king's son was a lot smaller than Elidore, but he guessed they were about the same age. The young prince was very friendly and greeted Elidore in the strange language he had heard the little men talking. The two boys rushed straight out to play. Elidore soon learnt enough words for them to understand one another and he learnt some wonderful games. Sometimes they played with beautiful golden balls which felt heavy and glittered as they rolled along the ground.

Elidore also learnt to ride one of the little horses. They found him one that was a bit sturdier than the rest, strong enough to bear his weight. It was a very different life from the one he knew. The people of this country didn't eat any kind of meat or fish, but lived on milk flavoured with saffron and a very light, delicious bread. And they behaved differently from people in the world he knew. They never swore or told lies. He sometimes heard them make disapproving jokes about the lies and treachery of the 'Big Men' in the world beyond the cave.

Elidore loved his new life, but after a while he began to miss his mother. One day he went to the king and asked permission to visit her. This was readily granted, though the king and the young prince begged him to come back soon. Elidore promised to return and the little men led him back to the cave, so that he could make his way home. His mother was very happy to see him and asked all about the life he was leading. He told her all about the country beyond the cave and his new friend and the games they played. When he described the golden balls, she became convinced that they were made of real gold. Then she said, 'You have found yourself a good life, Elidore, living in a king's palace. But I am poor and have no one to look after me. You could make all the difference to my life if you would bring just one of those golden balls for me.'

Elidore protested that the golden balls were not his to bring. But his mother pleaded with him and, because he loved her, he eventually agreed to do as she asked. Then he returned to his life on the other side of the cave, keeping company with the young prince until once again he became homesick and set off on another visit to his mother.

This time he slipped one of the golden balls into his pocket before making his way to the cave. As he was coming out on the other side, he heard the sound of running feet behind him. He started running towards his mother's cottage, but the feet were catching up with him. Reaching his mother's doorstep, he tripped and dropped the golden ball so that it rolled across the floor towards the corner where she was sitting. But at that moment the two little men who had been following rushed past him and grabbed the ball, chattering furiously and making angry faces at him. One of them grabbed the ball and they ran off with it.

Elidore was unhappy and didn't stay long visiting his mother. He was anxious to get back to his new life, but when he came to the place by the river where he had first seen the little men, he could not find the cave. Though he searched for it many times, he never found it and never got back to the land where he had spent such a happy time. Eventually, he gave up and returned to the monastery, to his studies, and became one of the monks. But he never forgot the time he had spent with the king's son and the little men. His stories about that time became well known throughout the land. People visiting the monastery would ask him to tell them. One day the Bishop of St David's, who was a learned man, came to visit Elidore and questioned him about the language he had learnt from the little men, observing that some of the words were very like Greek. But nobody ever solved the mystery of the country beyond the cave. And nobody ever found the way there again.

EURYNOME AND THE EGG
OF THE COSMOS
Greek Creation Myth

In the beginning was Chaos, an active and wild enlivening energy. Slowly forming came Eurynome, the Wide Wandering One. She rose from Chaos and searched for Matter on which to place her feet. She gave place to the sea and then to the sky, and so there was air and water coming from Chaos. Eurynome danced on her own upon the water and noticed that her dance caused a wind to follow behind. She whirled round and chased the wind, and when she caught it, she took it between her hands and moulded it, until it became Ophion, the great serpent.

Then Eurynome changed her shape and took on the form of a white dove. She nested over the water and in time gave birth to a large egg. She instructed Ophion to coil his body round the egg seven times until it split in two and hatched.

From this egg, the cosmos came! Mountains, forests, flowers, plains, deserts each fell into place. The sun and the moon dropped out, so that there was light, and so did the planets and the stars. All living creatures tumbled out of the egg, so that the land was formed and everything found its rightful place.

THE FLOWERING TREE
Native American

It seems that at one time the people were living scattered out all over the world, and each of them had heard about a very powerful person who lived in the river. It was said that this person could settle any problem, no matter what it was.

Because no one really wanted to admit to anyone else that they possessed problems, everybody had to sneak down to the river alone when they wished to hear this powerful person speak. And everybody did sneak down to the river to hear the powerful person, but no one ever spoke to anyone else about it.

Then one day a little boy and a little girl returned from the river. The little boy and the little girl began to talk to everyone about their journey.

'It was a very strange thing,' the children said.

'What was it that was so very strange?' the people asked as they gathered around the children, pretending they did not know.

'Have you not seen what is at the river?' the children asked.

'No,' the people all answered. 'What was it that you saw there?'

'Have all of you not sneaked down to the river, just as we did?' the children asked in surprise.

'Whoever said such a silly thing?' the people asked angrily.

'We did,' the children answered, becoming frightened.

'Never say such an awful thing again,' the people told them accusingly.

The children became even more frightened. They perceived that they were strangers, even to their own mothers and fathers.

This caused all the people to move away, leaving the little boy and the little girl alone upon the prairie. That night they were all alone and frightened. They cried, because everything seemed to be so terrible.

'Calm yourselves, my children,' a gentle voice suddenly said to them. The children looked to see who had spoken.

'Who are you?' the children asked.

'It is me, Old Man Coyote,' the voice said. As he spoke, Old Man Coyote entered the children's lodge and set down a bundle of firewood beside them.

'And it is me, Old Woman Coyote,' another voice said to them softly. She sat down and began to turn an arrow within her bow to make them a fire.

Soon there was a warm fire and there was light within their lodge. Sitting across the fire from them were an Old Man and an Old Woman.

'Who are you?' the children asked. They were now feeling better.

'We are your grandfather and your grandmother,' the Old Woman answered, offering the children some buffalo meat.

'And we are also the powerful person at the river,' the Old Man added, offering the children some sweet foods.

'But we saw only ourselves when we visited the river,' the little boy and the little girl said together.

'Yes, that is true,' the Old Woman and the Old Man answered together.

'I do not understand this,' the little girl said.

'How very strange,' the little boy said.

'The people have all visited the river as you did,' the Old Woman began.

'And they all saw only themselves, just as you did.' The Old Man finished the words.

'How very strange,' the little girl said.

'I do not understand,' the little boy said.

'They too thought it strange,' the Old Man answered.

'And they too did not understand,' the Old Woman answered.

'Were you also their reflections, as you were ours?' the little girl asked excitedly.

'And they did not trust their eyes,' the little boy said with excitement.

'Yes,' the Old Man said, 'you are right. Now you must find the people and offer them these gifts.

'What are these gifts?' the little girl asked.

'They are these two coyote robes,' the Old Woman answered. 'Tell them to put them on and they will not be hungry any more.'

And so the children did this. They found the people the next day and offered them the two coyote robes.

'What are these for?' the people asked. 'There are thousands upon thousands of these coyote robes to be had,' they laughed. 'What we need to satisfy our hunger are buffalo, not these silly robes.'

'Put them on,' the two children coaxed the people. And as they coaxed the people to put on the coyote robes, they spoke to them of their vision. But this only made the people laugh even harder.

Within this camp there lived two kind people. One was a man and the other was a woman. They were living together in the same lodge. These two kind people loved the little girl and the little boy, and wished to care for them. They both stepped into the circle of people and put their arms around the two children, adopting them.

'I will wear one of the robes,' the man said to the little girl.

'And I too will wear one of the robes,' the woman said to the little boy.

The children gave their robes to the man and the woman who had adopted them, and the man and woman put them on.

'There are buffalo to the North and to the South,' the man said to the people, because now he could see them.

'And there are buffalo to the West and to the East,' the woman said, because now she too could see them.

The people all became excited, because suddenly they too could see the buffalo.

'Let us hunt them in the North,' some of the people said.

'No,' others quickly shouted. 'The buffalo are much fatter in the South.'

'No! No!' still others argued. 'They are bigger in the West.'

'No! No!' the rest of the people said angrily. 'The best ones of all are to the East.'

'Please! Please! Do not fight among yourselves,' the man, woman, little boy and little girl pleaded. 'You are only tricking yourselves. Put on the coyote robes and you will understand.'

But the people were very angry, and they would not come together in a circle to counsel.

'Kill these trouble-makers,' the people shouted. And they rushed in all together upon these four who were sitting in the middle of the camp circle. But when they reached the centre of the camp circle, they discovered that the little boy and the little girl had become a flowering forked tree. They quickly looked for the man and the woman who had adopted the two children, but all they found of them were their tracks. They were the tracks of two mountain lions. These tracks were leading to the North.

The people were so angry they struck at the flowering tree.

'Let us follow the two lions and kill them,' the people decided together. They followed the tracks to the North to find them. They ran and ran, until suddenly the tracks of the two lions became the tracks of four lions. These led the people in a great circle back to the flowering tree.

The people sat down together around the tree because they were so tired, and they began to talk to one another.

'Why are we doing this?' some of them asked the others.

'We do not really wish to hurt or kill anything,' said some others.

'Then why were you running?' asked still others.

'We were only following you,' those spoken to said in amazement. And they all began to laugh.

Then the people all heard singing and they looked up. There, sitting in the North, they saw a white coyote and he was singing. They also looked to the South, and sitting there was a green coyote. She too was singing. Then they looked to the West, and sitting there was a black coyote and he was singing. Finally, they looked to the East, and sitting there was a gold coyote and she was singing.

The people sat there quietly all together and learned these four beautiful songs. They were the songs of four lions. Then the people looked all around and saw that each of them was wearing a coyote robe. They put their arms around each other and began to dance toward the flowering tree together in a great circle. The people were happy.

FOREVER-MOUNTAIN
Japan

Long ago, a famous wrestler called Forever-Mountain was on his way to wrestle before the Emperor. He was swinging his huge legs and humming a tune, feeling pleased with himself. Beside a river he saw a young woman walking ahead of him, carrying a pitcher of water on her head. He said to himself, 'If I don't tickle that girl and make her laugh, I'll never forgive myself!'

So he crept up behind her and did just that. The girl did laugh, but then she brought down her arm and caught his hand against her body. He could not get free from her hold. The more he tried to tug his hand away, the more she laughed. She walked him up to the top of the mountain. At last he was begging her to set him free, telling her that he was on his way to an important wrestling competition at the Emperor's palace.

At that the young woman, whose name was Maru-mei, laughed even more and said, 'Poor little Sumi wrestler! Do you want me to carry you up the mountain?'

By this time all he wanted was to get away from the girl and forget he had ever seen her. Crossly, he asked what she wanted of him. She said that she wanted to help him because, if she could manage him so easily, what would happen if he came up against a really strong man? Forever-Mountain turned pale at the thought. At her suggestion, he agreed to stay for three months at her mother's house, so that her mother and grandmother could work on him.

She led him over the mountain and into a small valley where she stopped in front of a farmhouse, saying, 'Grandmother will be sleeping now, but here comes Mother, bringing our cow in from the field!'

He looked at an older woman walking round the house and saw that she was carrying a cow in her arms. She explained that she did this so that the cow would not hurt her hooves on the sharp rocks of the mountain path. Then she asked her daughter who the young man was. The young woman replied, 'He says he is a Sumi wrestler, but he is very weak. I brought him home to work with us.'

Her mother looked him over and said, 'He'll need some good food to build him up. When he gets stronger, he can help Grandmother around the house.'

Then the grandmother came out of the house. She tripped over the root of a tree that was growing near the door and complained that it was always tripping her up. Then she pulled the tree up by its roots and tossed it to the side of the path. The Sumi wrestler almost fainted with terror. The grandmother said, 'Poor young man, he really is very feeble. We had better put him straight to bed so that he can rest.'

Next morning the work began. The three women gave Forever-Mountain some well-cooked rice, but ate theirs hard and almost raw. Day by day they prepared his rice with less water. They made him do the work of five men around the farm and in the evenings he wrestled with the grandmother. At first she could easily throw him up in the air and catch him without losing her smile. He soon forgot that, beyond this valley, he was one of the finest wrestlers in Japan. Day by day he grew stronger until a time came when he could stamp his foot and the people in the village below would remark that it was late in the year for thunder.

At last he was strong enough to pick up a tree and throw it. Then, one evening when he was wrestling with the grandmother, he held her down for half a minute. The three women applauded and all agreed that it was time for him to go and wrestle in front of the Emperor. They told him to take the cow with him, sell her and buy the broadest, most handsome belt he could find. They said, 'Wear it for us in the wrestling contest!'

Thanking them, he slung the cow on his shoulder and walked over the mountain. He sold her in the market place and bought the most beautiful, silken belt he could find. Then he went to join the other wrestlers, waiting for the contest to begin. He found them all boasting and eating enormous bowls of rice, but he just sat quietly and waited.

When the people of the court were all gathered and the Emperor took his place, ready for the grand event, Forever-Mountain and another wrestler were called in. As they faced one another, Forever-Mountain stamped his foot with a sound like thunder. The first wrestler turned pale and retired and so did five more. After that, Forever-Mountain took care to stamp lightly, then picked up each wrestler that challenged him very gently and placed him in front of the Emperor with a polite bow. There was simply no contest.

Because people enjoyed the national sport of wrestling and wanted to see real fights, Forever-Mountain was then presented with a huge bag of gold, on one condition: that he withdraw permanently from all competition. He returned to the valley with his bag of gold and asked Maru-mei to marry him. They built a beautiful house for themselves, while the mother and grandmother lived on in the farmhouse close by. Having proved himself the champion of all Japan, Forever-Mountain was happy to spend the rest of his days with Maru-Mei, farming the land and raising a family.

THE GREAT WHITE BIRD

Bushmen, South Africa

A hunter lived on the edge of a great African forest. One day he was out hunting and stopped to drink from a pool. As he bent down over the water, he saw the reflection of a great white bird flying overhead. He leapt to his feet, intent on following the bird, but it was already disappearing over the trees.

The hunter followed the direction the bird had taken until he came to the far side of the forest. By then the bird was long out of sight, but still the hunter travelled on, determined to catch up with it. He asked all the people he met if they had seen a great white bird. Some hadn't seen it at all. Others said, 'Oh, yes, we saw it only yesterday. It went that way. Keep going and you will probably catch up with it.'

He kept travelling on, leaving his home and family and all that was dear to him far behind. There was never any doubt in his mind that he had to follow the white bird until he caught up with it. Weeks passed, months passed and, eventually, years. Every now and then he encountered someone who said, in answer to his question, 'Oh yes, we have seen the bird. It flew past yesterday!' He was always just too late to catch a glimpse of it.

Travelling on across the great continent, he grew tired and eventually old, but he never gave up. At last he came to the tallest mountain in Africa. The people who lived near the mountain said, 'The white bird lives at the top of the mountain – up there, beyond the snow line!'

Then the hunter knew that he was near his journey's end. If only he could get to the top of the mountain, he would see the white bird. He started to climb. The path became steeper and steeper. He was becoming breathless, but kept on climbing until he was just below the snow line. Then he stumbled and fell. Realising that he could go no further, he threw himself on the ground and cried out like a child, 'Oh, Mother, I have failed!'

As he lay there, he heard a voice say, 'Look up!' He looked up and saw a white feather drifting down towards him, out of the red evening sky. Reaching up, he caught it in his hand and died content.

THE HANDLESS MAIDEN

German Fairytale, Grimm

Once upon a time a miller and his wife had an only daughter. The times were bad, and the mill did not prosper. They became poor and hungry.

One day when the miller was walking in the forest to cut wood, he met an old man, whom he had never seen before. The old man said, 'Why do you trouble yourself with chopping wood? I can make you rich if you will promise me what stands behind your mill.' The miller thought to himself that the only thing behind his mill was an old apple tree. So he said, 'Yes,' and concluded the bargain.

When he got home, his wife said, 'Where has all this money come from? Suddenly, all the bowls and drawers in the house are filled with money.' 'That,' said the miller, 'is no problem. I met an old man in the woods an hour ago, and he promised to make me rich if I just let him have whatever was at the back of the mill.' The wife said, 'You fool, our daughter was out there sweeping this afternoon.'

So one day the devil, for that is who the old man was, comes to get the miller's daughter. The father has by now explained to his daughter that he has sold her, and she is to stand there and wait for the old man when he comes to fetch her. But overnight it turns out she has drawn a circle around herself. When the devil comes, he cries out, 'I don't like circles! I hate circles! No more circles! Tomorrow I'll come again. Make sure there are no more circles.' The father says, 'But what can I do?' 'Tie her hands in front of her so she can't draw. Or else I'll take you.'

So the father goes to his daughter and says, 'I'll have to tie your hands together.' 'Whatever you say, Father,' answers the daughter. So he does.

But when the devil comes again in the morning, it turns out she has been weeping all night on her hands, and they have been washed clean by her tears. The devil is furious. 'Hands washed by water! I don't like washed hands, especially hands washed by tears. I don't like tears. No more washed hands, understand?' 'But what can I do?' says the father. 'Cut her hands off, or else I cannot have her.'

The miller is horrified. He says, 'How can I cut off the hands of my own child?' The devil answers, 'If you do not, you are mine, and I will take you yourself away.'

So the father goes to his daughter and tells her what the devil has said, and asks her to help him in his trouble and to forgive him for the wickedness he is about to do her. She replies, 'Dear Father, do with me what you will – I am your daughter.' And her father cuts her hands off.

But when the devil comes again in the morning, it turns out that the daughter has been weeping all night on the stumps where her hands have been cut off, and the stumps are washed clean of blood. And the devil says, 'Oh, the hell with it. I can't deal with this. You can keep her.'

And the devil goes off.

The miller now says to his daughter, 'I have received so much good through you that I will care for you most dearly all your life long.'

But the daughter answers, 'Here I cannot remain. I will wander forth into the world, where compassionate men will give me as much as I require.' And she asks her father to tie her arms behind her back and departs on her journey.

In time she arrives at a royal garden where she sees a tree standing which bears beautiful fruit. But she cannot enter, because the garden is ringed with water. She is tormented with hunger. So she kneels and prays for help. An angel appears, who makes a passage through the water, so that she can pass. So she goes into the garden, but all the pears are numbered. She steps up to the tree and eats one to appease her hunger, but no more. The gardener who watches over the tree sees her, but does not interfere because he is afraid of the strange figure with her.

The next morning the king found that a pear was missing and asked the gardener where it was. The gardener explains what he had seen, and the king says, 'I'll watch tonight.' So he does. He sees her cross the water, again accompanied by a shining being. She comes to the tree and reaches up her face, her arms tied behind her back, and eats a pear. The king comes out and speaks with her. He likes her, and in time they are married, and the king has a pair of silver hands made for her.

After a year has gone by, the king has to go away to war. Soon after, his wife has a baby boy, who is named Rich in Sorrow. The king's old mother sends a message to the king with the joyful news, but on his way the messenger sleeps, and while he is sleeping the devil changes the letter for another one that announces that the queen has brought a changeling into the world. The king is much troubled by the letter, but writes back to his mother that she should take great care of the queen until his return. But again the devil intercepts the letter, substituting one that says the queen and the child are to be put to death, and the tongue and eyes of the queen sent to the king as proof that it has been done. The old mother is horrified at these orders and says to the young queen, 'I cannot let you be killed as the king commands, but you must remain here no longer. Go forth with your child into the wide world and never return.' So she binds the child on to the queen's back, and the poor wife goes away, once more into the wilderness of the forest. Meanwhile, the old queen arranges for a calf to be killed and its tongue and eyes sent to the king.

The last part of the story runs in parallel for seven years. The king comes home and realises what has happened, and goes out into the world to search for his wife and child. The queen wanders in the forest with her little son. One day she comes to a spring and wants to drink, but is afraid to do so lest the child should fall into the water. Then the water slowly rises, she looks again and gets so thirsty that she leans forward and the child slips from her arms and falls in. In despair she begins to cry out and to walk round. An old man comes up and says, 'Take the child out!' But she says, 'I have no hands!' The old man repeats, 'Take the child out!' Then she plunges her arms into the water, and suddenly, where there had been stumps only, living hands grow, and she is able to seize hold of the child and lift it out.

At last, after his seven years of searching, the king finds his way to the little cottage named 'Here all dwell free' where the queen has found shelter. Exhausted with his searching, he lies down, covers his face with a napkin and falls asleep.

His wife and child return, and find him asleep on the floor. The napkin has fallen off his face, and the queen says to the boy, 'Rich in Sorrow, the napkin is falling off your father's face. Pick it up and cover him carefully.' The child does as he is told, and the king, who heard in his sleep what passed, lets the cloth fall again from off his face.

The queen says once again to her son, 'Rich in Sorrow, the napkin is falling off your father's face. Pick it up and cover him carefully.' At this the boy becomes impatient, and says to his mother, 'How can I cover my father's face? I have no father on earth. I have learned the prayer, "Our Father, which art in Heaven," and you have told me my father is in heaven. How can I talk to this wild man? He is not my father.'

As he hears this, the king raises himself up and asks the queen who she is. She replies, 'I am your wife, and this is your son, Rich in Sorrow.'

At that the king is glad and full of joy. Then he sees her human hands and says to her, 'But my wife has silver hands.'

Which may be the end of the story…or maybe not.

SESSION PLAN FOR ENACTMENT OF *THE SNOW QUEEN* AT CENTRAL SCHOOL OF SPEECH AND DRAMA

Photographed by Camilla Jessel Panufnik

FOCUS

Arriving to the room and each other
Checking in with your body – what you need to let go of the journey through the London cold
Is there warmth in this place?

WARM-UP

Passing a rhythm round the circle
Opening and closing the body
Stretching and moving out into the room
Meeting others and moving with them

VOICE WARM-UP

Finding a hum, extending into vowels and adding consonants
Passing a sound round the circle
Gobbledy gook conversations with one or two others

BRIDGE IN

Using movement, sound and material, create two lands either side of the room
One has the qualities of summer, the other has the qualities of winter
Explore the relationship between ice and warmth as a whole group

MAIN EVENT

Telling of *The Snow Queen* story
Selection of roles
Placing the locations of the story in the room
Story enactment using sound, movement and minimal words
Reflection on the character you have played
De-role from character back to self

BRIDGE OUT

Spelling 'Eternity' from ice – full group sculpt
Personal reflection – patterns of warmth and ice in your life?
Working in movement, show the hot/cold quality that you are working on in your own life – how can your partner respond to this?
Work both ways
Time to talk in twos
Time to talk in the larger group

GROUNDING

Moving to your own rhythm
Preparing to take the warmth but prepare for homewards journey through London cold
Final name call round the circle

ENACTMENT OF *THE SNOW QUEEN*

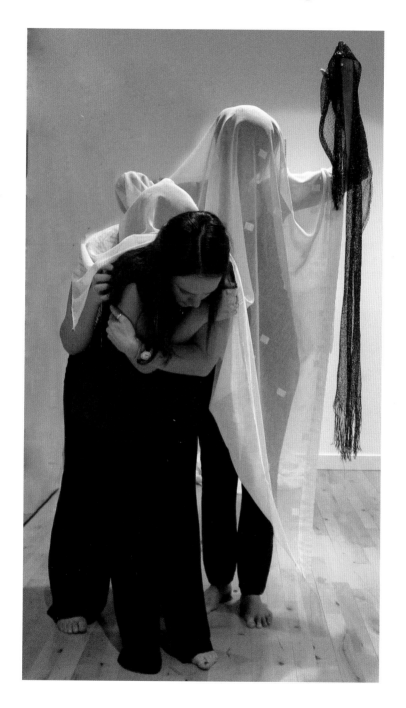

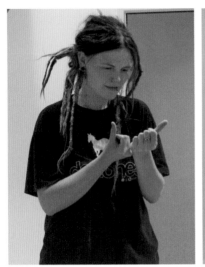
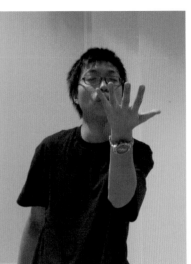
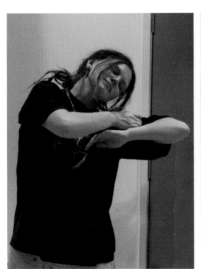
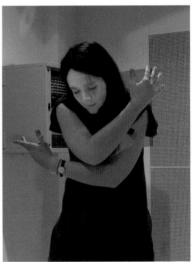

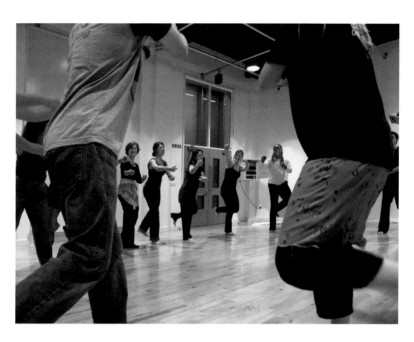

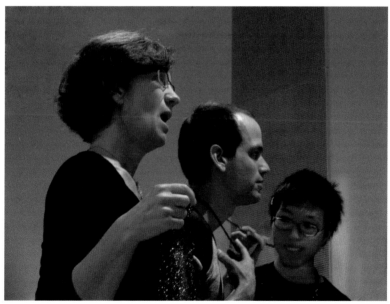

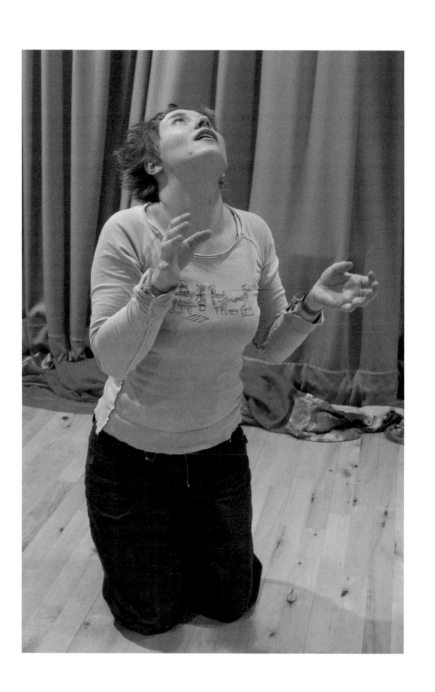

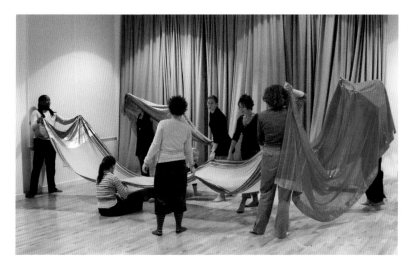

The warm land

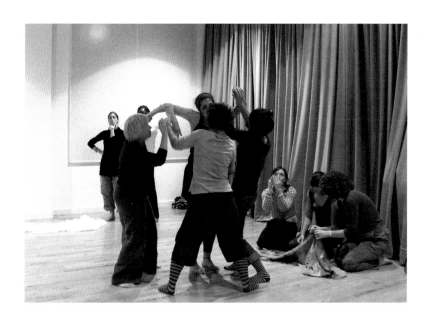

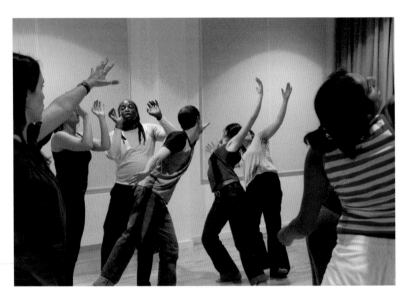

The cold land

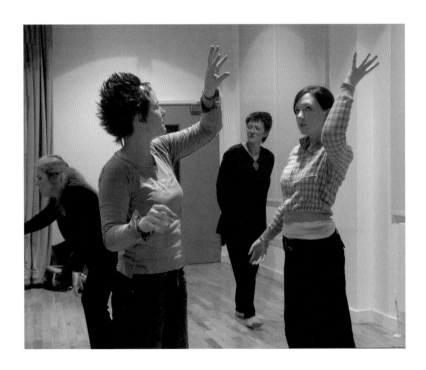

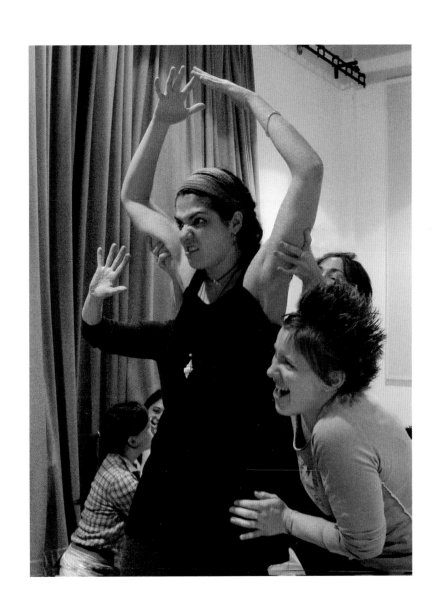

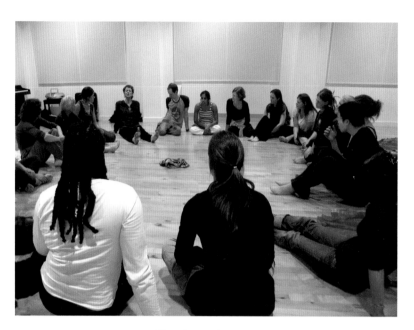

Listening to the story

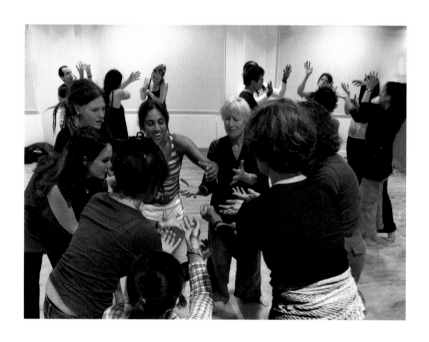

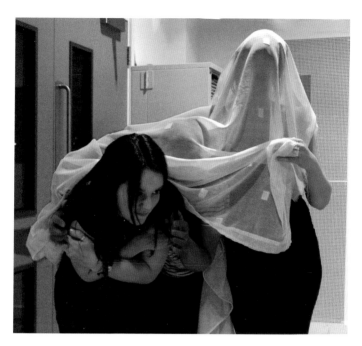

Kay and the Snow Queen

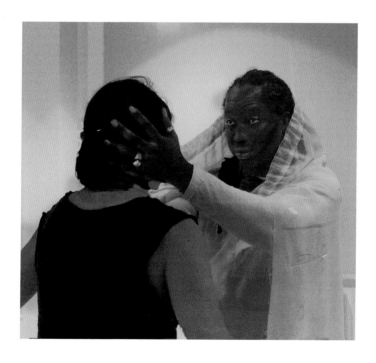

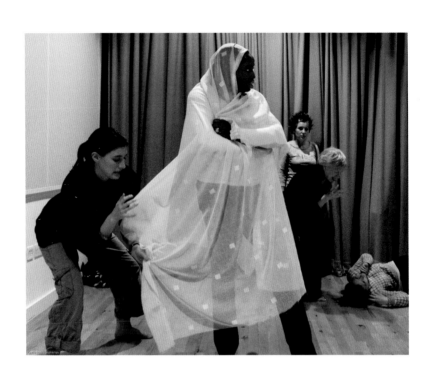

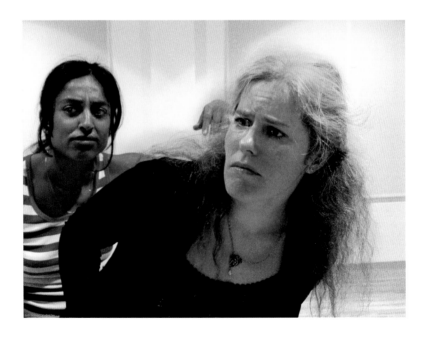

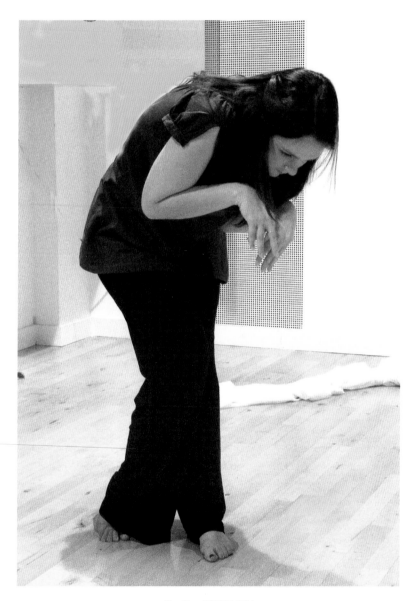

Spelling ETERNITY

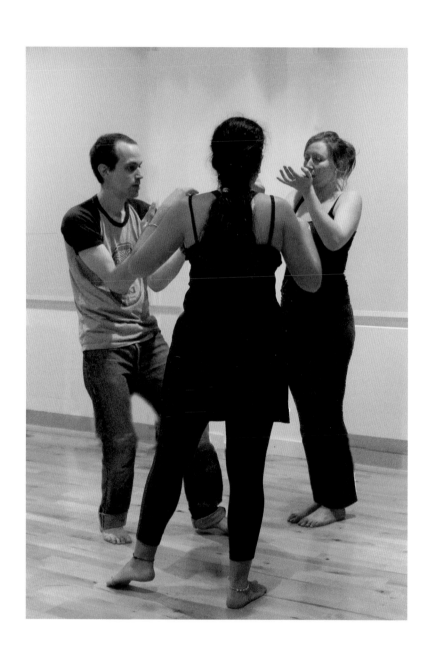

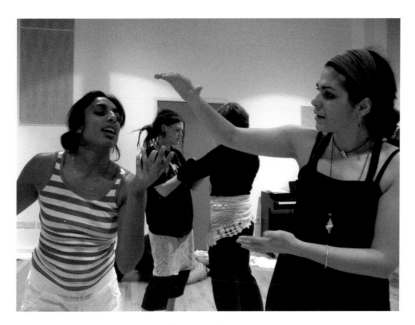

Energy exchange

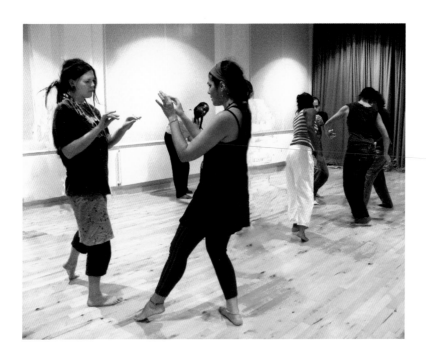

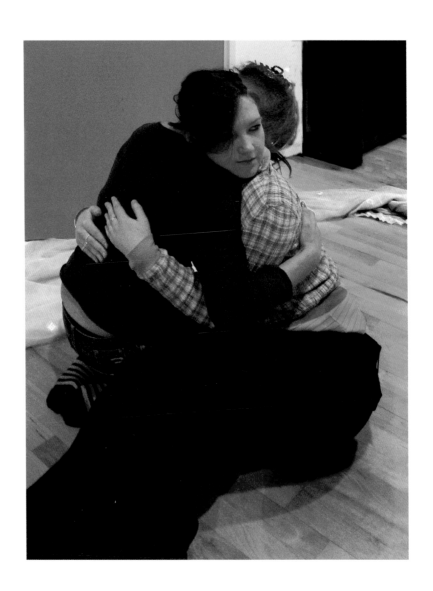

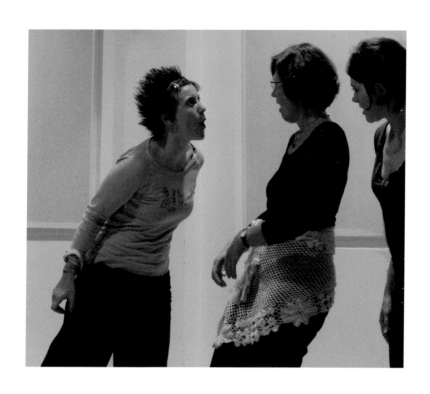

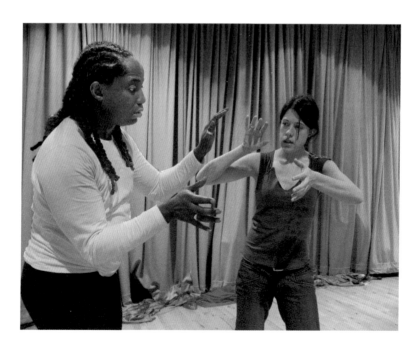

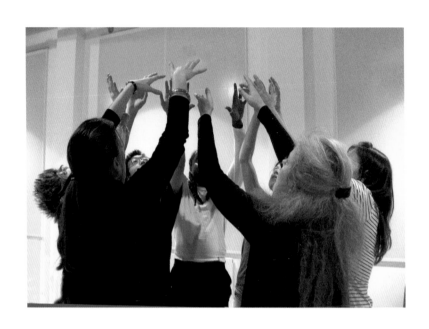

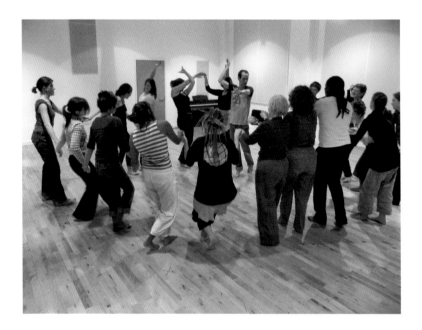

THE HEALING HERB
Sesame Original

A traveller was walking along a country road. He had been travelling restlessly for a long time, looking for something, though he did not know what he was looking for.

One morning he found himself outside a walled garden. He was curious to see the garden, but there seemed to be no way in. There was a vine growing round the wall. Searching among the leaves and branches of the vine, he found a door handle. He tried the handle and the door opened. Inside, the traveller found a beautiful garden filled with bushes and trees, flowers and butterflies and singing birds. But the garden was heavily overgrown with brambles and weeds of every kind. He heard the sound of digging and scraping a little way off. Making his way through the bushes, he found a gardener struggling to clear the weeds from a patch of ground. He offered to help the gardener and they worked together all day. When at last all the weeds were cleared, they came upon a wonderful, scented herb. The gardener thanked the traveller for his help and gave him a piece of the herb. The traveller said goodbye and went on his way.

He hadn't gone far when he came upon a frog panting at the side of the road, parched and exhausted after straying too far from the river. As he bent over the frog in concern, a piece of the herb fell on it. The frog immediately sat up, refreshed and quite well, thanked the traveller and hopped on its way. A little further on, he heard some yelping and a dog limped out of the bushes on three paws, holding up the fourth, which was mangled from being caught in a trap. Remembering what had happened with the frog, the traveller took a piece of the herb and rubbed it on the dog's paw. The wound healed over immediately and the dog went on its way with no trace of a limp.

The man travelled on and a few days later he arrived at the outskirts of a town. Here he met a weeping woman with a dying child in her arms. The man offered her a piece of the herb and she administered it to the child. The child recovered immediately.

The man travelled on and used the herb to help everyone who needed it. Very strangely, however much he used it, the herb did not fade or get any smaller. Whenever he gave away a piece of it, it grew back to its original size and shape. The traveller became known as a healer, and people in all sorts of trouble began to seek him out. At length he realised that the herb was the thing he had been looking for on his travels.

THE HOLY GRAIL
British Legend

As a boy, Parsival was kept from the world by his mother. His father, a Knight in the court of King Arthur, had died in battle before Parsival's birth, and her son was all that she had left, so she did not want to risk him. She kept him hidden in the depths of a forest and denied him knowledge of his noble birthright to be a knight.

One day, Parsival heard a great clatter of iron and a cavalcade came by, and he saw Knights in armour which sparkled in the sun. Parsival believed he was seeing God's angels and he knelt before them. When the Knights told them who they really were, it awoke his calling to destiny, and he begged his mother to let him go to the King's court. His mother reluctantly gave her consent, but set Parsival off, dressed in fool's clothing, so that no one would take him seriously. However, they did make him a Knight of the Round Table.

After many adventures, he arrived at the castle of the nobleman Gorneman, who took Parsival in and taught him the rules of chivalry. The fool's clothing was taken away, and Gorneman taught him about courtesy and the ethics behind courtesy. He told Parsival that he must never lose his sense of shame, he must never importune elders with foolish questions and he must always remember to show compassion to those who suffer. Although Parsival carefully memorised these fine words, he didn't truly understand them.

In due course, Parsival's travels took him to a wasted land, where everything was barren and there was deep famine. Looking for shelter, he came to a castle where he found the King – a fisherman – was gravely ailing, thrashing about in an agony from a wound in his groin. The Fisher King was waiting for a Knight who would ask him the necessary questions which would bring about the healing that was so needed. His hope was raised when Parsival arrived. However, when Parsival saw the sick king on his bed, he forgot about showing compassion to those who suffer and held back the question that roused his curiosity, for fear that he would shame himself. The outer form of Gorneman's advice was strong in his mind, and all he could think of was the requirement that he should not importune elders with foolish questions.

During the evening meal, a slow procession of people entered the room, accompanied by the sweetest sounds of celestial music.

A girl entered, carrying the Grail between her hands, which gave forth a burst of heavenly light. When the Grail passed close to the guests, each one was served with meats, varied dishes and drinks, according to his most secret desires and according to what he asked. The rich Fisher King watched Parsival with great sadness as the Holy Grail came to him, but Parsival, struck dumb by timidity, postponed the questions that burned on his lips. The Grail passed him by. Led to his room, he fell asleep and during the night there was a great clap of thunder, and the castle vanished. Parsival rode off into the wilderness, into the cold, grey dawn with the words 'You've failed' echoing in his mind. Baffled and heavy-hearted, he followed a trail through gloomy woodland until he met a woman, who, on hearing he had visited the Grail Castle but had said nothing about the King, in the presence of the Grail, was aghast. 'Did you not see his suffering? Could you not find it in your heart to ask the cause of such great pain? The Grail has vanished again and all hope with it. The land must still lie wasted.'

In shame, Parsival continued on his way. One day he encountered the ugliest and most hideous female figure he had ever seen, mounted on a mule and carrying a whip in her hand. She too reviled Parsival for not having asked about the Grail. Parsival remonstrated, 'I didn't know, no one told me, I was told not to ask questions.' The ugly hag scoffed, 'And do you only do what you're told? Is obedience the only wisdom? Has the heart no knowledge of its own?' Then she added harshly, 'And do you know, your mother's dead! You killed your own mother and she died of a broken heart.'

For five years, Parsival wandered aimlessly through the land. He had lost all remembrance of God, a thing so important to a Knight of the Round Table. He fought endless battles and proved himself over and over as a powerful warrior. However, these victories did nothing to pacify his feelings of guilt and emptiness.

Lost and battle-weary, he found his way to the hut of a holy hermit. He fell at the hermit's feet weeping. He asked to make confession about the years he had forgotten God. When the hermit asked him why this had happened, Parsival told him of his visit to the King and his failure to speak, and how this had weighed so heavily on him that he had abandoned faith. The hermit granted him absolution, and Parsival again set out on his way. He was still not yet ready to know exactly what he must do, but he had acquired hope once more. After this he met many more adventures, but always the Grail dominated his thoughts.

One day, lost in a mysterious wood, Parsival prayed to God to lead him to the Grail Castle. Towards evening, the castle appeared out of the mists. Once again Parsival was led to the Grail King, seated now on a purple couch. Parsival viewed the sick King with compassion, sorrowing because of the King's profound suffering. He humbly gave an account of his long adventures and spoke openly of his failures. Then he lifted a gentle hand to soothe the pain that seared across the wounded man's brow. In the immense, attentive silence of the hall, he heard himself whispering, 'What ails thee, King?' At these tender words, colour began to come back into the Fisher King's face. In the same instant, the whole chamber glowed luminously with the radiance of the Holy Grail. Parsival stood transfixed. He then turned to the King again and asked, 'Whom does the Grail serve?' When the King heard these words, he arose, miraculously restored to health and strength. The land too was restored, the whole kingdom rejoiced and a great springtime of joy and life began.

THE HYMN OF THE PEARL
Gnostic Story, Middle East

When I was a little child and dwelt in the kingdom of my Father's house and delighted in the wealth and splendour of those who raised me, my parents sent me forth from the East, our homeland, with provisions for the journey... They took off me the robe of glory which in their love they had made for me, and my purple mantle that was woven to conform exactly to my figure, and made a covenant with me, and wrote it in my heart that I might not forget it: 'When thou goest down into Egypt and bringest the One Pearl which lies in the middle of the sea which is encircled by the snorting serpent, thou shalt put on again thy robe of glory and thy mantle over it and with thy brother, our next in rank, be heir to our kingdom.'

I left the East and took my way downwards, accompanied by two royal envoys, since the way was dangerous and hard and I was very young for such a journey... I went straightway to the serpent and settled down close by his inn until he should slumber and sleep so that I might take the Pearl from him... I clothed myself in their garments, lest they suspect me as one coming from without to take the Pearl and arouse the serpent against me. But through some cause they marked that I was not their countryman, and they ingratiated themselves with me and mixed me (drink) with their cunning, and gave me to taste of their meat; and I forgot the Pearl for which my parents had sent me. Through the heaviness of their nourishment I sank into deep slumber.

All this that befell me, my parents marked, and they were grieved for me... And they wrote a letter to me, and each of the great ones signed it with their name.

'From thy father, the King of Kings, and from thy mother, mistress of the East, and from thy brother, our next of kin, unto thee our son in Egypt, greeting. Awake and rise up out of thy sleep, and perceive the words of our letter. Remember that thou art a king's son: behold whom thou has served in bondage. Be mindful of the Pearl, for whose sake thou has departed into Egypt. Remember thy robe of glory, recall thy splendid mantle, that thou mayest put them on and deck thyself with them and thy name be read in the book of heroes and then become with thy brother, our deputy, heir in our kingdom.'

Like a messenger was the letter... It rose up in the form of an eagle, the king of all winged fowl, and flew until it alighted beside me and became wholly speech. At its voice and sound I awoke and arose from my sleep, took it up, kissed it, broke its seal, and read. Just as was written on my heart were the words of my letter to read. I remembered that I was a son of kings, that my freeborn soul desired its own kind. I remembered the Pearl for which I had been sent down to Egypt, and I began to enchant the terrible and snorting serpent. I charmed it to sleep by naming over it my father's name, the name of our next in rank, and that of my mother, the Queen of the East. I seized the Pearl, and turned to repair home to my father. Their filthy and impure garment I put off, and left behind in their land, and directed my way that I might come to the light of our homeland, the East.

My letter which had awakened me I found before me on my way; and as it had awakened me with its voice, so it guided me with its light that shone before me, and with its voice it encouraged me, and with its love it drew me on... (Then, as he approached his homeland his parents sent out to him his robe of glory and his mantle.) And I stretched toward it and took it and decked myself with the beauty of its colours. And I cast the royal mantle about my entire self. Clothed therein, I ascended to the gate of salutation and adoration. I bowed my head and adored the splendour of my father who had sent it to me, whose commands I had fulfilled as he too had done what he had promised... He received me joyfully, and I was with him in his kingdom.

IN THE BEGINNING
Native Australian

In the beginning was Dreamtime. The spirits lived on earth with the animals and people. The Great Spirit made all things.

In the beginning the earth was completely flat and the sky was so close to it that there was no room for birds to fly, nor for animals and people to grow to their full size. There were no lakes, no billabongs. There was only one pool. It was so well hidden that the Great Spirit himself had forgotten it was there.

It so happened that by chance the Great Spirit came upon the pool. He drank its waters and bathed in it. When he stepped from the pool, the magic of the pool was in him. For the first time he saw that the earth was too close to the sky. That there was no space for birds to fly, and that man and animals could not grow to their full size.

So, lifting up his arms, he pushed at the sky. Men saw him and they pushed too. As they pushed, mountains arose from the surface of the earth and the Great Spirit became bigger. Now there was space for birds to fly, and man and animals could grow to their full size. Some of the waters of the pool rose up with the sky and became clouds. Rain fell, flowers grew and green grass and rushes.

The people praised the Great Spirit.

The Great Spirit made himself a sky camp. He saw that his work was good and he was content.

When the people slept, the flowers had seen the Great Spirit's camp. They wanted to be with him in the sky. They crept up into the sky. When the people woke in the morning, they were sad to see that there were no flowers. Children ran about searching for them. Bees were unable to make honey. Butterflies were tired and fell to the ground.

At last the old men of the tribe decided to seek out the Great Spirit in his sky camp. They wanted him to help them. The old men climbed for many days. The jagged rocks cut into their feet. At last they reached the top of the mountain. They could see the sky camp.

The Great Spirit listened to their request. He was troubled. He did not want his sky camp to be empty of flowers; neither did he want the people on earth to be unhappy. He thought for a long time. At last he said to the old men, 'Pick as many flowers as your arms can hold. Take them back to earth and scatter them about your camps. They will take root and flourish. In the hottest days of summer they will die, but they will return in the spring.'

The old men picked the flowers, as many as they could carry. They made their return journey. They scattered the flowers on the bare brown earth. They took root and flourished. Children laughed again. The young girls danced and sang, twining the flowers in their hair. Bees made honey. Butterflies alighted on flowers and spread their wings.

On the hottest day of the summer the flowers withered and died. In the spring the flowers returned again, just as the Great Spirit had said. The people were happy. The Great Spirit watched from the sky and was glad to see their joy.

INANNA IN THE UNDERWORLD
Ancient Sumer

The Queen of Earth and Heaven inclined her ear to the Great Below. She heard the sound of grieving. Her sister Ereshkigal, Queen of the Underworld, was grieving for the death of her husband Gugulanna, the Great Bull of Heaven.

Inanna said, 'My sister is grieving. I will go to the Underworld and grieve with her.'

She dressed herself in the seven mē, the garments of her power. She placed the crown of the Steppe on her head. She tied her little lapis beads around her neck. She let the double strand of beads fall to her breast. She wrapped the royal robe about her body. She daubed her eyelids with the ointment that is called 'Let him come, let him come!' She tied about her chest the breastplate that is called 'Come, man, come!' She slipped the gold ring over her wrist, and in her hands she held the lapis rod and line, all symbols of her power.

Inanna set off on her journey to the Underworld and her faithful servant Ninshibur went with her. When they came to the entrance of the Underworld, Inanna turned to Ninshibur and said, 'I will descend alone to the Underworld. Wait for me here. If I do not return within three days, set up a lament for me. Beat your drum in the assembly places. Go to the temple of the god Enlil and say to him, "Oh Father Enlil, do not let your daughter be put to death in the Underworld." If Enlil will not help you, go to Nanna's temple and ask his help. If Nanna will not help you, go to the temple of Enki. He knows the food of life and the water of life. Enki will not let me die.'

Then Inanna embraced her servant Ninshibur and left her, walking alone to the gates of the Underworld. Before the first gate, she called to Neti the gatekeeper to open the gates.

Neti called back through the first gate, 'Who are you that stands at the Gate of the Underworld?'

She replied, 'I am Inanna, Queen of Heaven and Earth. I come for the funeral rites of Gugulanna. I come to mourn with my sister Ereshkigal, your Queen.'

Neti said, 'Stay there while I speak with my Queen.' He left Inanna standing at the first gate and went down to Ereshkigal, standing before her and saying, 'Inanna is standing at your gates, dressed in the seven *mē*, garments of her power. She has come to mourn with you.'

Ereshkigal frowned and she told Neti to bolt all the gates of the Underworld. As Inanna passed through each gate, he was to take from her one of the garments of her power. 'Let the Holy Priestess of Heaven enter my kingdom naked and bow low!'

Neti returned to Inanna and opened the first gate, saying, 'Come, Inanna. Enter!' As she stepped through the gate, he took from her head the great crown of the Steppe.

Inanna asked, 'What is this?' Neti replied, 'The ways of the Underworld are perfect and must not be questioned!'

At each of the gates he took one of her garments, until she came to the seventh gate and he took the last garment. Inanna passed through the seventh gate into the great hall of the Underworld, naked, with her head bowed.

She was surrounded by the *Annuna*, judges of the Underworld, and her sister Ereshkigal fastened the eye of death upon her. Inanna was turned to a corpse, a piece of meat, and hung on a hook on the wall of the Underworld.

For three days and three nights, her servant Ninshibur waited at the gates of the Underworld. On the third day, when Inanna had not returned, Ninshibur took her drum and set up a lament for her in the holy places. She circled the houses of the gods, coming to the temple of Enlil. Standing before him, she said, 'Oh Enlil, do not let your daughter be put to death in the Underworld. Do not let Inanna die!' But Enlil replied, 'Those who go to the Underworld do not return. I cannot help Inanna.'

She went to the temple of Nanna and said, 'Oh Father Nanna, do not let your daughter be put to death in the Underworld!' But Nanna replied, 'I cannot help Inanna. Those who go to the Underworld do not return.'

Finally, Ninshibur stood before Father Enki and begged him to save Inanna. Enki, who loved her, took a piece of dirt from under his fingernail. From it he fashioned two little creatures, neither male nor female, a *kurgarra* and a *galatur*. He gave the food of life to the *kurgarra* and to the *galatur* he gave the water of life. Addressing them, he said, 'Go to the Underworld. Enter through the gates like flies. You will find Ereshkigal grieving, moaning like a woman about to give birth, her breasts uncovered and her hair hanging like leaks. When she cries, "Oh oh, my inside," you must say, "Oh, oh, our inside!" And when she cries, "Oh, oh, my outside," you must say, "Oh, oh, our outside!" Whatever she cries, cry with her. She will be comforted and will offer you a gift. Whatever she offers, refuse it. Then she will ask you what you want. Ask for the piece of meat that hangs on the wall. Sprinkle on it the food of life and the water of life. Then Inanna will arise.'

And so it was. The *kurgarra* and the *galatur* went like flies through the gates of the Underworld. They found Ereshkigal and grieved with her. When she cried, 'Oh, oh, my inside,' they cried, 'Oh, oh, our inside.' When she cried, 'Oh, oh, my outside,' they cried, 'Oh, oh, our outside.' Whatever she cried, they echoed it. At last Ereshkigal was comforted. She said, 'Because you have comforted me, I will give you the water gift. I will give you the river in flood.' But they replied, 'We do not want the river in flood.' She said, 'I will give you the grain gift. I will give you the fields in harvest.' But they replied, 'We do not want to fields in harvest.'

Then Ereshkigal said, 'What do you want?' They replied, 'We want only the corpse that hangs from the hook on the wall!'

So the corpse was taken down and laid before them. The *kurgarra* sprinkled it with the food of life and the *galatur* sprinkled it with the water of life. Inanna arose and walked towards the gates of the Underworld.

Then the *Annuna*, the judges, said, 'If Inanna returns to the world above, she must find someone to take her place in the Underworld! The *galla*, demons of the Underworld, will go with you and bring someone back in your place!'

So the *galla*, the demons, went with her through the gates. At the last gate they found Ninshibur, her faithful servant, waiting. They said, 'Walk on, Inanna. We will take Ninshibur in your place!' But Inanna said, 'No, you shall not have Ninshibur! She is my faithful servant and she saved me. I will not give you Ninshibur.' And the *galla* said, 'Walk on, Inanna. We will come with you.'

As they went towards the city of Uruk, they came to a shrine by the road. Inanna's son, Shara, was waiting there for his mother, dressed in sack cloth, with ashes on his head. The *galla* said, 'Walk on to your city, Inanna. We will take Shara!' But Inanna said, 'No! You shall not have Shara! He has grieved and waited for me. I will never give you Shara!' And the *galla* said, 'Walk on, Inanna. We will come with you.'

When they came to Uruk, they came upon Inanna's husband, Dumuzzi, dressed in fine raiment, seated on a throne and playing his shepherd's pipe. When Inanna approached, he made no move to greet her. She fastened the eye of death upon Dumuzzi and said, 'Take him!'

The *galla* went to seize Dumuzzi, but he screamed for help to Utu, the god of justice, and Utu turned him into a gazelle. The *galla* could not hold him and he ran out of the city to the home of his sister Geshtinanna, who loved him. She hid her brother in a sheepfold, but the *galla* found him and bound him, preparing to take him away.

His sister Geshtinanna wept for Dumuzzi. Standing before Inanna, she pleaded with her to be allowed to go to the Underworld in her brother's place. Then Inanna wept in sorrow for Dumuzzi, the shepherd she had loved and married. She said to him, 'You will have to go, but only for half the year. Your sister Geshtinanna will take your place after six months, but when she returns, you will have to go again. And so it will be for the rest of time.'

And so it has been, from that day to this.

IRON HANS

German Fairytale, Grimm

A King's palace was close to a great forest. One day he sent a huntsman into the forest to shoot deer and the huntsman did not come back. Another huntsman went to look for him, and then another, but neither returned. The King sent a search party into the forest, but they could find no trace of the huntsmen or their dogs. After that the King forbade anyone to enter the forest.

Time passed and a hunter came from far away asked the King for permission to go into the forest. The King tried to dissuade him, but the man was determined and eventually the King gave his consent. Near the edge of the forest, the hunter's dog picked up a scent and the hunter followed it to the edge of a deep pool. He saw a hand and a long, hairy arm reach out of the pool and pull his dog under the water.

The man returned to the court and asked for three men to go back with him into the forest, bringing with them buckets to empty the pool. At the bottom of the pool they found a wild man lying in the mud. He was brown as rusty iron with hair all over his face and hanging down to his knees. They tied him up and carried him back to the palace where the King ordered him to be put in an iron cage in the courtyard. The door of the cage was locked and the King forbade anyone to open it, on pain of death. The key was given into the Queen's keeping. From that day, people walked and hunted safely in the forest.

One day the King's eight-year-old son was playing in the courtyard with a golden ball. He let it fly into the cage and the wild man caught it. When the boy asked him to return the ball, the wild man said, 'Not unless you open the door of the cage.' The boy refused, saying the King had forbidden it. Next day the boy returned to the courtyard and the wild man asked him again to open the cage, but again he refused. On the third day, when the King and his court were out hunting, the scene was repeated and the boy told the wild man that he couldn't open the cage because he didn't have the key. The wild man told him it was under his mother's pillow.

The boy fetched the key and unlocked the door of the cage. The wild man stepped out, gave the boy his golden ball and started running towards the forest. The boy called after him, 'Wild man,

wild man, don't leave me here. They'll kill me for letting you out!'
The wild man picked him up, placed him on his shoulders and ran
with him into the forest.

When the King got back, he saw that the wild man had gone.
The Queen went to look for the key and found that it had been
taken from under her pillow. The boy was nowhere to be seen. They
searched all over the palace and into the forest, but could find no
trace of him.

The wild man, whose name was Iron Hans, ran deep into the
forest with the King's son on his shoulders. At length he stopped in
front of a wooden hut. He lifted the boy down and made a bed of
moss in the hut for him to sleep on. He promised that he would look
after him well, adding that he had some treasure hidden away that
would one day belong to the boy.

Next morning Iron Hans showed the boy a golden spring near
the hut and told him to watch over it, making sure that nothing fell
into the clear water. Iron Hans himself would be gone all day, but
would return with food in the evening.

The boy sat by the spring and watched over the clear pool. Now
and then he saw a golden snake or a golden fish in the water. He
made sure that nothing fell in. Suddenly, his finger began to hurt
and, without thinking, he put it in the water to cool. Then he saw
that his finger had become golden. He tried to wipe off the gold but
could not. When the wild man returned in the evening, the boy hid
his hand behind his back. Iron Hans immediately knew what had
happened and said, 'You have dipped your hand in the water. Don't
do it again.'

Next day the boy was left to guard the pool again and felt his
finger hurting. This time he ran his hand through his hair, but one of
his hairs fell into the pool. He pulled it out of the water, but the hair
had become golden. Again the wild man knew what had happened.
He warned the boy that if he defiled the pool again, he would not be
able to stay in the forest.

On the third day the boy was sitting by the pool and leant over
the water to look at his reflection. All his hair, which was long, fell
forward into the water, and when he raised his head it glittered like
the sun. He tied a handkerchief around his hair so that the wild man
would not see it, but Iron Hans was not deceived. He told the boy
that he must leave the forest and make his own way in the world.

But if he was ever in trouble, he could come to the edge of the forest, call 'Iron Hans' three times and ask for help.

The King's son left the forest and walked into a nearby town, looking for work. He could find none that he was skilled enough to do. Eventually, he came to the palace of another King and was given work, fetching wood and water and sweeping the ashes. He wore a hat at all times to hide his bright, golden hair. One day he was asked to wait on the King at table. The King asked why he wore a hat and he said it was because he had scurf on his head. He was promptly dismissed from the table and the kitchen, but the cook persuaded the gardener to give him work out of doors.

One warm day he was working in the garden and took off his hat to cool his head. The sunlight fell on his golden hair and a bright shaft of light was reflected into the Princess's bedroom. She looked out and, seeing the boy with golden hair, she called him and asked him to bring her a bunch of flowers. He picked some wildflowers, tied them with string and took them to her room. As he walked through the door, the princess snatched off his hat and his golden hair tumbled out. She gave him a handful of gold coins, but, having no interest in coins, he gave them to the gardener's children to play with.

Next day the Princess asked him for another bunch of wild flowers. She tried to snatch his hat again, but this time he prevented her. Even so, she gave him another handful of coins, which again he gave to the gardener's children. On the third day the same thing happened.

The country was at war and the King feared defeat because his enemy was powerful. The young man asked for a horse, saying that he wanted to go and fight for the King, but they would only give him an old horse that limped. He rode the old horse to the edge of the forest and called for Iron Hans.

When the wild man appeared and asked what he wanted, the young man asked for a sturdy horse to ride into battle. Iron Hans fetched a prancing charger and a troop of Iron Men from the forest to fight on his side. The young man rode to the war with his Iron Men and saved the day. The King told his daughter about the strange knight who had ridden to their rescue with a troop of soldiers and she wanted to know more about him, but they had all galloped off and the King had no idea who they were.

Then the King proclaimed a festival, to be held over three days, with his daughter throwing a golden apple every day. He and the

Princess thought the strange knight might come and compete. The young man went back to the edge of the forest and called Iron Hans, telling him that he wanted to catch the Princess's golden apples. The wild man gave him a chestnut horse and a suit of red armour, and he took his place among the other knights, caught the first apple and rode away. Next day he came in white armour on a white horse, caught the second apple and rode away. On the third day the King gave orders that the knight who caught the apple must be not be allowed to escape.

Riding a black horse and wearing black armour, the King's son caught the apple on the third day. As he was riding off, one of the King's men chased after him and nicked his leg with the tip of a sword. The young man's horse reared and his helmet flew off as he galloped away, revealing his bright golden hair.

Next morning the Princess asked the gardener if his young man was working in the garden that day. The gardener replied that he was, adding that he had astonished his children by showing them three golden apples. Then the Princess asked her father to send for the gardener's boy and, as he walked in, she pulled off his hat, revealing his golden hair.

The King asked if he was the knight who had won the three golden apples and he replied that he was, taking them out of his pockets. He told the King that he was also the knight who had fought for him, displaying the wound on his leg to prove it. When the King praised and thanked the young man, asking if there was anything he could do to reward him, the young man promptly replied that he could give him his daughter in marriage.

So a wedding was arranged. The young man's parents were among the wedding guests, most happy to be reunited with their lost son. When the festivities were in full swing, another King walked into the hall with a huge retinue, embracing the Prince and announcing himself as the wild man, Iron Hans. He said, 'I was under a spell, but you have set me free. Now all my treasure is yours!'

JUMPING MOUSE

Native American

A small mouse lived on the plains with his family. Their whole life was taken up with continually searching out grass blades and sage leaves, all the time, every day, so that they could eat delightful things. Mouse, however, could hear a sound, in the distance, always there. When he asked the others about it, they scorned him, for they could not hear anything. They thought he was strange and mad.

One day Mouse happened across Brother Raccoon, and Mouse asked him about the sound. Brother Raccoon knew exactly what it was and said that, if Mouse liked, he could show him. They travelled until they came to a huge rushing-along river, full of eddies of currents and life energy. Raccoon introduced Mouse to Brother Frog, who sat midstream, as if he had been waiting. Frog welcomed Mouse and said, 'Brother Mouse, if you want good medicine, then crouch down low and leap up high and see what you will see.' So Mouse crouched down low and leaped up high, and just for a moment, when he was high in the air, he caught a glimpse of the Sacred Mountains. Then he landed, splash, back down, into the river and he was wet all over. He was furious with Frog! But Frog told him to remember what he had seen, and he gave Mouse a new name. The name was Jumping Mouse.

Jumping Mouse returned to his family. He was river-wet and they thought some creature had eaten him then spat him out, not finding him tasty enough to nourish them. They would not believe anything he said about rivers and frogs or mountains. So Jumping Mouse decided to leave them to it, and go and find the Sacred Mountains on his own.

Travelling by night, for fear of eagles, Jumping Mouse travelled until he reached a lush area of sage. A fat mouse lived there and made him welcome, showing him the delights of the sage patch. Sage Mouse told Jumping Mouse that while there certainly was a river, there were no Sacred Mountains, and even if there were, why would anyone want to go there with the eagles always overhead? Just stay put! So for a while Jumping Mouse stayed, but then he remembered what he had seen. So he set out again, and, overhead, the eagles watched.

He travelled by night and eventually arrived at a place full of berry bushes. Hidden there was a sick creature, lying on the ground, groaning in pain. He told Jumping Mouse that he was Brother Buffalo and he could be healed, but only if he had the eye of a mouse, and everyone knew there was no such thing as a mouse. Jumping Mouse saw that Brother Buffalo was a very great creature, and offered his mouse eye. As soon as he spoke this, the eye left him and Buffalo was healed. Buffalo thanked Jumping Mouse and said he might travel onwards to the Sacred Mountains, underneath his belly, so that the eagles would not see him. Jumping Mouse scuttled across the prairie, so close to the great hooves of Brother Buffalo, terrified of being crushed, yet both safe and protected.

At the foot of the Sacred Mountains, Buffalo told Jumping Mouse he could take him no further, but soon he would meet Brother Wolf who would be his guide. Jumping Mouse waited till a creature came to him. 'This must be Wolf,' he thought. 'Greetings, Brother,' said the wolf. 'I am…? I am…em…I am… *Who* am I…? Oh yes, I am a…' Jumping Mouse could see that this fine animal was suffering because he could not remember who he was. Perhaps the eye of a mouse would help? As soon as he said this, his eye left him, and immediately Wolf remembered. He told Jumping Mouse he was the guide to the Sacred Mountains, and he led Jumping Mouse up the steep slopes. Soon they came to a lake, where Wolf told him the whole world and everything about everything could be seen, but, of course, Jumping Mouse had no eyes. Then Wolf told Jumping Mouse he must leave him there, completely on his own.

Jumping Mouse was quite alone. Nearer and nearer he could feel the eagles closing in on him. Nearer and nearer, until, THUD, all went dark. They had Jumping Mouse.

Then a strange thing happened, for as morning came Jumping Mouse woke up. He could see blurred shapes and sizes and colours, and he could hear a voice which called to him, 'Jumping Mouse, do you want good medicine? If you do, crouch down low and jump up high and trust the wind.' So Jumping Mouse did this, and the wind lifted him higher and higher. 'I am afraid!' shouted Jumping Mouse, and the voice shouted back, 'Trust the wind.' Jumping Mouse did this, and when he opened his eyes, he could see everything. The higher he flew, the clearer he could see. Jumping Mouse saw the river and Frog way below. Frog called to him, 'Jumping Mouse, do you want a new name? No longer can you be called Mouse for now you can fly. Your new name is Eagle.'

KAANG

Bushmen, South Africa

You see, creatures did not always live at the surface. At one time they lived Deep-Down with Kaang, the Lord of Life and of all creatures. Although they lived in darkness, the only thing that mattered was the light of their oneness with each other. There was no fear, for there was perpetually enough of what was needed, and Kaang planned to make a world above and to fill it with all that had been created below.

So Kaang made a tree with roots going down and branches going up. He told the people and the animals to choose what they most loved from below and take this above, up through the roots of the tree. And he told the women and the men that when they made the new place, they must never light fire. If they did, what was precious would be lost and spoiled, and this was agreed.

Taking their gifts and placing them above, the animals and people lived the first day, but when the sun went down, fear arrived in their hearts because they could no longer see. The darkness grew deeper and in the cold blood of panic, someone shouted, 'Let us make our own light.' In this way, fire was made and the people were warmed and could once again see. But when the animals saw the fire, they pulled back and withdrew.

Further and further from humankind they fled. Since that day Kaang's people no longer understand the darkness or speak easily with animals. No longer can they be one, and the friendship so dearly held between them has been lost. For people cannot tolerate anything which they cannot immediately see or quickly understand. And that is how it was, and, of course, still is.

KING LAURIN

Austria

Long ago, the King of the Alps lived inside one of the mountains of the Tirol. His palace was underground and his name was King Laurin. King Laurin was said to own all the gold and silver in the world. He also had a daughter who was young and beautiful, unlike her father, the goblin King, who was short and fat with a bulbous nose and looked as old as the mountains themselves.

King Laurin's daughter loved flowers and was sad that none grew in her father's snowy kingdom. She longed particularly for roses, roses the colour of sunrise and sunset. When she told her father of her longing, he gave orders for a rose garden to be created with a crystal roof so that the roses would have the light and warmth they needed to grow strong and fragrant. People in the valley were amazed to see the snowy mountains suddenly glowing with rosy colour. They called it the Alpen glow.

King Laurin was a kind goblin. He was merry and full of tricks. He sometimes went down into the valley and visited people, surprising them with his generosity and his pranks. Stories were told about his visits and this is a story that mothers in that valley still tell to their children.

A poor cobbler was living in the valley. His wife had died, leaving him with three young boys to look after. Their names were Fritzl, Franzl and Hansl. The hut they lived in was so small. It had only one room with a cobbler's bench, a hearth for cooking, a big straw bed and a table and stools. The cobbler fed them with whatever he was given in addition to his payment. When he mended the farmer's shoes, they had butter and milk. When he worked for the butcher, he came home with meat for a stew. He would cook up the meat with vegetables and herbs and take the lid off the pot with a great flourish, saying, 'Today we eat the good Schnizzle, Schnozzle and Schnoozle!' It was nonsense, but somehow the stew tasted better because of it.

A hard time came when the country was at war. The men in the farms and villages were called away to fight. Their women and children were left behind to look after themselves as best they could and everyone was short of money. People stopped having their shoes mended, just walked around with broken heels and flapping soles, and the poor cobbler struggled to feed his children. In summer it wasn't so bad as he could grow a few vegetables, but by the time winter arrived their situation was desperate. On Christmas Eve the cobbler went down to the inn, hoping to find someone who needed their shoes mending. While he was gone, the boys went out and gathered a few sticks for a fire. It was crackling in the grate by the time their father came home with good news. Soldiers were marching into the village, the inn was full and soon he would have plenty of work. Soldiers always needed their boots mending.

Meanwhile there was no supper. Their father told the boys to bolt the door, stoke up the fire and keep warm in the bed until he returned. 'And don't open the door to anyone!' he said.

Then he picked up his bag of tools and was gone. The three boys cuddled up in the big straw bed and the night grew colder and colder, the wind whistling and roaring around the hut. Suddenly, they heard a loud knocking. Franzl reminded them that their father had told them not to open the door. But Fritzl couldn't resist peeping out. On the doorstep he saw a little man no bigger than Hansl pounding on the door. Now they could all hear him calling, 'Let me in! Let me in!'

Fritz's brothers tried to stop him, but he couldn't leave anyone shivering on the doorstep in such weather. He drew back the bolt and in burst the oddest little man. He had a peaked cap on his head, big ears and a bulbous nose, and his teeth were chattering. He stepped inside and shook his fist at the boys, saying, 'Ach, so you keep me waiting? Want to keep all the good food and warmth to yourselves? Greedy boys!'

Fritzl tried to tell him that they weren't greedy, that there was no food, but the little man wasn't listening. He just said, 'Greedy boys, you've eaten it all. Well, at least you can warm me. Roll over. Give me half the quilt! Come on, make room!'

He jumped into the bed and pulled half the cover over himself. Fritzl tried to get in beside him but the little man said, 'Nah, nah, I'm going to have your place in the bed.' Then with one foot he kicked poor Fritzl right across the room, saying, 'If you want to keep warm, turn cartwheels. Turn them fast!'

Not knowing what else to do, Fritzl did just that. He turned cartwheels round the room. As his feet swung over his head, things began to fall out of his pockets. And behind him he left a trail of oranges and sweets, wrapped in gold and silver paper. At last he stopped and stood up, gaping at the all good things scattered across the floor.

Now the little man dug Hansl in the ribs and said, 'Time for you to do some cartwheels. Out you go – turn cartwheels and keep warm!' Hansl was kicked out of bed and then he was turning cartwheels across the floor. From his pockets fell Christmas buns and delicious iced cakes.

The angry little man pushed Hansl, the youngest, out of the bed and said, 'Turn cartwheels!' Fritzl protested that Hansl was too small, that he couldn't do cartwheels. The little man said, 'Then pick him up by the ankles and shake him!'

Fritzl and Franzl picked up their little brother by the ankles and shook him gently. From his pockets poured gold and silver pieces, scattering over the floor and rolling into the corners. Hansl cried, 'Put me down! Put me down!' Then all three boys began to gather up the good things on the floor and pile them on the table, shouting with excitement. When at last they turned towards the bed, it was empty. The little man had disappeared and the quilt lay in a heap on the floor.

At that moment the door opened and in came their father, carrying bread and milk and meat for a Christmas stew. Seeing all the good things piled up on the table and the gold coins on the floor, he said, 'Whatever is happening?' When they told him, he said, 'Aren't we the lucky ones? I always thought it was just a story. Now I see it's true that good King Laurin likes to visit at Christmas time, to play his tricks and share his treasure.'

'Yes, but he was such an ugly little man,' said Hansl. 'He dug us in the rubs and took all the bed to himself!'

'That is the King,' their father said. 'He likes to play at being fierce, but look how kind he is! And now, tell me, what shall we eat tonight?'

The three boys replied with one voice 'The good Schnizzle, Schnozzle and Schnoozle!'

KOROZUKA
Japan

Late one night a priest and his servant lost their way in the marshes. The wind was rising and the night was cold. Suddenly, in the distance they saw a light. They made their way towards it. The light was coming from the window of a hut. As they approached, they heard the noise of a spinning wheel and the sound of singing.

They approached and knocked on the door. The singing and spinning stopped. An old apple-cheeked woman came to the door. They asked for shelter for the night. The old woman asked them in. They sat on the floor and she went back to her spinning. For a long while the old woman eyed them as she moved her fingers on her wheel. The priest could see she was not at rest, but troubled and full of disquiet. He began to speak to her of enlightenment. At length he won her attention. She stopped spinning and listened. Her mood became harmonious and she was at peace with herself.

She offered the priest and his servant food. They were welcome to rest the night in the hut, but first she would gather some sticks for a fire. The night would be cold. While she was gone, she warned them that on no account must they open the door at the other end of the hut. The priest and servant said they would not and settled down to sleep.

The priest was soon asleep. The servant tossed and turned. He was curious about what lay behind the forbidden door. He got up and crept towards the door. He put his hand on the handle and listened. Not a sound. The priest slept. At length he opened the door. He let out a long cry. Before him was a room filled with the flesh and bones of men. He realised that the old woman was a man-devouring demon. He woke the priest, pointing to the room. He ran out on to the marsh.

Under a full moon the old woman was dancing and singing as she collected sticks. Never before had she known such peace of mind. Suddenly, there before her was the servant, wild with fear. At once she knew her trust had been betrayed. He had looked behind the door. Her expression changed and she became the devouring demon she had always been. Her hands became claws. The servant ran to the priest. The demon followed into the hut. Demon and priest confronted each other.

THE LION, THE YOUNG MAN AND THE BLACK STORM TREE

Bushmen, South Africa

One day a young man of the early race went out hunting. He was hot. He came to a pool, lay down and fell asleep.

A lion comes to the pool for water. He sees the young man, goes silently to him and drags him towards a tree. Afraid that if he stirs the lion may kill him, he keeps still, pretending to be dead.

The lion places him in the fork of a black storm tree – a tree which has no thorns and bears lovely yellow flowers. The lion decides to go to the pool and drink before it eats the young man. So, fixing the young man still more firmly into the fork of the tree, it sets out towards the water. It turns round, goes back to make sure the young man is firmly there.

The lion has indeed fixed the young man so firmly that a sharp bit of wood protrudes into his back, hurting him intensely. He has been crying quietly to himself and the tears have started running down his face. When the lion reaches him, it immediately sees the tears that have started running down the young man's cheeks. It gently licks them away. Then the lion goes to the pool. It will return. The moment the young man is convinced that the lion has gone for a while, he jumps up and runs back to his own community. He runs in a zig-zag because he knows that because the lion has licked away his tears it will come back for him. He does all he can to put the lion off the scent.

He tells his people that there is a lion coming after him. He begs them to wrap him in the tough skins of the hartebeest.

His mother and the people did as he asked. He was their hearts' young man.

The lion comes, looking for the young man. It stands quite still. The people attack the lion with arrows and spears. It stays quite still and says, 'I have come for the young man whose tears I have licked and whom I must find.'

The people offer the lion children and even a young woman instead, but the lion refuses to be sidetracked.

By nightfall the frightened people realise they can do nothing. It is between the lion and the young man.

Despite his mother's pleading, they take the young man from the covering. The lion recognises him and kills him. It speaks to the people, saying, 'Now I have the young man whose tears I licked, he is mine and I am his. Now you may kill me.'

The people killed the lion. It lay beside the young man. The people were at peace.

THE LITTLE EARTH COW
Fairytale from Alsace

A poor man had two daughters, Amy and Gretel, whose mother died when they were young. Their father remarried and their stepmother became jealous of Gretel, who was the darling of the household. She longed to get rid of Gretel, but dared not harm her openly. Instead, she made friends with Amy, Gretel's older sister. She encouraged Amy to hate her sister. Together, the stepmother and Amy plotted to get rid of Gretel by taking her on a picnic and abandoning her in the forest.

But Gretel was listening outside the door and heard them making their plan. Frightened, she ran to her grandmother's room to ask for her help. The grandmother said, 'Don't tell anyone else what you have heard. Just collect some sawdust and keep it in your pocket. When they send you to gather firewood, leave a trail of sawdust on the path. Then you will be able to find your way back through the forest and home.'

Next day a picnic was announced and everything went according to the plan Gretel had overheard. She was sent off to gather wood for a fire in the part of the forest where the trees were thickest. When she turned to walk back with the firewood, there were trees all round her and every direction looked the same. But she was able to follow the trail of sawdust, as her grandmother advised, and soon came back to the edge of the forest. As there was no sign of her sister and stepmother, she returned home by herself.

The stepmother managed to cover her surprise when Gretel walked in. However, it wasn't long before she and Amy were plotting another expedition. Gretel overheard them and ran to her grandmother, who advised her this time to fill her pocket with chaff. The place chosen for the picnic was even deeper in the forest and they disappeared while she was gathering firewood, but again she left a trail of chaff and was able to make her way safely home.

When a third picnic was arranged, Gretel could not find her grandmother to ask for help. She remembered about the sawdust and the chaff, but could find neither. Instead, she filled her pockets with hempseed. She felt safe enough when they sent her off to gather wood. However, when she turned to look for the trail of hempseed, there was no trail to be seen. The birds had eaten up every last seed and Gretel was completely lost in the middle of the forest.

She ran in every direction looking for a way out. Soon it began to get dark and still she was surrounded by trees. Then she climbed into a very high tree, thinking she might be able to see a village or even a house in the distance. All she could see was a little column of smoke coming from a clump of trees in the distance. She climbed down and walked in the direction of the smoke until she came to a tiny house, the home of a little Earth Cow.

When Gretel knocked on the door, the Earth Cow said, 'I shall not let you in unless you promise to spend your life here with me and never tell anyone about me.'

Gretel was so relieved to be offered shelter that she willingly gave her promise. The little Earth Cow opened the door and said, 'You are welcome to my home. All you have to do here is milk me in the morning and in the evening. Then you can drink my milk and do whatever you like all day while I am at pasture. I will bring you silk and velvet so that you can make all the pretty clothes your heart desires. But you must take care never to tell anyone about me. Even if your own sister comes to the door, don't let her in. And don't betray my existence, for if you do I will lose my life.'

So the little Earth Cow gave her milk and Gretel shared her home. In the daytime the Earth Cow went out to pasture, returning in the evening with silks and velvets for Gretel. Time passed and Gretel made herself a lot of pretty clothes and came to look like a princess.

Having managed to lose Gretel in the forest, her stepmother was happy. But after a while Amy began to miss her sister. One day she decided to go into the forest and see if she could find any trace of Gretel. After walking a long way she, too, was lost among the trees and climbed the same tall tree to look for a way out. She caught sight of a plume of smoke and walked towards it until she found herself outside the little Earth Cow's house. Knocking on the door, she was greeted by her sister, dressed in the most beautiful clothes and looking happy. The Earth Cow was out at pasture and Gretel was on her own.

Gretel welcomed her sister. When Amy asked whose house it was, she first said that it belonged to a wolf and then to a bear. Amy didn't believe her. She went on questioning her, promising not to tell anyone her secret. At last Gretel was convinced by her sister's sweet manner and revealed that the house belonged to the little Earth Cow. 'But you must never betray me!' she said.

Amy promised Gretel that she would tell no one. She asked Gretel to show her the way out of the forest and went home. Of course, she told her stepmother all about the visit, describing how happy Gretel looked and how beautifully she was dressed. Again the stepmother became jealous and said, 'Next week we will go and find Gretel. We will bring the Earth Cow home with us and eat it.'

The Earth Cow knew everything at a glance when she got back to her house. She said sadly, 'Alas, dear Gretel, what have you done? You have let your sister in here and told her about me. Now they will kill me and treat you even worse than before.'

Gretel couldn't bear to see the Earth Cow look so sad. She started to cry, saying how sorry she was. And she couldn't bear it if the Earth Cow had to die. The little Earth Cow tried to comfort her and said, 'What has happened cannot be undone. But I can tell you how you can make things come right in the end. When the butcher slaughters me, stay there and cry. He will ask what you want him to do. Ask him to give you my tail and one of my horns. Then cry some more and ask him to give you my Earth Cow's shoe. When he has given you these three things, dig a deep hole in the ground and plant first my tail, then my horn on top of the tail and, last of all, my shoe on top of the horn. Do not return to the place where they are planted for three days. On the third day they will have grown into a tree. This tree will bear the most beautiful apples ever seen, both in summer and winter.'

It turned out exactly as the little Earth Cow had foreseen. Gretel's sister told the stepmother everything. She brought her to the little house in the forest and they took Gretel and the little Earth Cow home with them. The butcher was called to kill the Earth Cow. Gretel stood by and cried while this was happening and, at her request, she was given the tail, the horn and the shoe. She planted them and a tree grew that bore the most beautiful apples.

One day a nobleman whose son was very ill passed by and saw the tree. He asked for some apples to take home to his son. The stepmother and Amy went to pick apples for him, but the tree pulled its branches away and would not yield its fruit. It would only give its apples to Gretel. Then the nobleman asked Gretel if she would come with him and give the apples to his son. When she gave him one of the apples, the young man tasted it and was immediately cured. He rose from his sick bed and, charmed by Gretel, fell in love with her. They were married and from that moment Gretel had a happy life.

LOKI AND BALDUR
Norse Myth

Baldur was the son of the god Odin and the goddess Frigg; a handsome young man, greatly loved and admired by the people. Loki, the Trickster God, was jealous of Baldur because he was not liked so much.

One night Baldur dreamt that he was going to die. Terrified, he told his mother Frigg about the dream and she, wishing to protect him, went to all the animals and creatures of the Earth, to all the trees and rocks and even the vegetables, getting them to promise that none would harm her beloved son. Then, to reassure him, she told Baldur what she had done.

Baldur, being young and boastful, began to strut a little and challenge people to see if they could harm him. He was full of confidence, knowing that his mother had magical powers and that he was protected.

Seeing this, Loki hated and envied him more than ever. He made up his mind that somehow he would find a way to hurt Baldur and, if possible, get rid of him. Disguising himself as an old woman, he went to visit Frigg, and asked after Baldur's health, listening very carefully as she told him what she had done to protect her favourite son. By careful questioning, he discovered that she had thought of almost everything, but had not yet asked the help of the mistletoe that winds itself around the trunk of the oak tree.

Now Loki saw his chance. Immediately after his conversation with Frigg, he threw off his disguise and went into the forest in search of a tree with mistletoe growing around it. Finding an oak tree, he climbed up into its branches and cut himself a piece of the mistletoe, stripped off its leaves and carved it into an arrow.

He ran straight to the village, holding the arrow in his hand. He found Baldur standing there, still defying anyone who wanted to throw things at him. Baldur's blind brother, Hod, was sitting quietly on the edge of this scene. Loki went up to Hod and asked him why he wasn't throwing things at Baldur like other people. Hod replied, 'I have nothing to throw. And, even if I had a branch or a stone in my hand, I can't see to take aim.'

Loki said, 'You shouldn't miss out on the fun. See, I will help you!' He put the arrow of mistletoe in Hod's hand and steered it, helping him to throw the arrow.

It struck Baldur through the heart and he fell to the ground, dead. Everyone who saw it gasped and looked to see where the arrow had come from. Seeing Loki's triumphant face, they knew who had murdered Baldur.

THE MAGIC DRUM
Canada, Inuit

An old man and woman had a beautiful daughter. She had refused all proposals of marriage. Eventually, two brothers came from a great distance, and the moment they entered her parents' igloo, she was attracted to them. She followed them outside, and when she saw them reach for two skins they had left at the door, she realised what made them different from her other suitors. They were white bears.

They seized hold of her and dragged her over the ice. When they came to a hole in the ice, they pulled her into it and on through the water, under the ice. When they came to another hole in the ice, they left her. The woman sank down and down until she found herself walking on the ocean floor. Looking around, she saw darkness in one direction and light in another. She reasoned that the darkness must be the north and colder, so she walked towards the light and the south.

As she walked, she found herself surrounded by tiny sea animals that nibbled at her body, tearing away strips of her flesh. Little by little she was devoured until only her skeleton remained. Still she walked towards the light. At last she came to a crevasse and was able to climb out on to the ice. Then she sat down and remembered her home and how her parents always kept the larder stocked with food. Realising she must do something to look after herself, she gathered some ice and built a small igloo with a storage platform for food. Then, feeling very tired, she fell asleep in her ice cabin. Her last thoughts were that she must somehow find some skins to make clothes and a sleeping bag.

When she awoke and went outside, the woman found a big igloo like her father's standing in front of her own and, beside it, a freshly killed caribou. She realised that her last thoughts before falling asleep had come true. She skinned the caribou, made a sleeping bag and some clothes, and put the meat on a storage shelf. Then she ate a good meal and slept. After that everything she thought about before going to sleep was there for her to find in the morning. She had a comfortable life except that her flesh, having been eaten by the sea creatures, could not be replaced. She remained a walking skeleton.

Every day the skeleton woman went exploring over the ice. Sometimes she saw young men out hunting for seals, but though she longed for company, they always fled in fear when they saw her approaching. Two of these young men had an old father whose wife had died some years ago. They didn't take him on their hunting expeditions, but on the day they saw the skeleton woman, they told him about her. They said, 'She seemed to want to be friendly, but we were afraid and ran away.'

The old man said that, as he was old without much longer to live, he would go on his own the next day to look for the skeleton woman. He found her sitting in the entrance to her igloo and she invited him in. The igloo was brightly lit with stone lamps. She offered him a meal and a sleeping bag and they both slept soundly. Next morning the young woman who was a skeleton asked the old man to make her a small drum. He made one from caribou skin and handed it to her. She blew out the lamps, took the drum in one hand and began to beat a rhythm. As she beat the drum, she sang. The drum grew larger, filling the air with its sound, and the woman danced in the dark. At last the music and the dance came to an end and she lit the lamps. Standing before him, the old man saw a beautiful young woman, dressed in the finest clothes.

Then she put out the lamps and danced again, beating the drum. After a while she asked him if he was all right as he sat there in the dark. He replied that he felt fine and when she relit the lamps he was a handsome young man. The drum magic had worked on them both.

That is how the young woman who had not wanted to marry found herself a husband.

When the couple walked into his home, his sons did not recognise their father. They said their father had walked away into the north and had not returned. The man told them that he was their father. He had been old and she had been a skeleton, but both were now young and she was his wife.

MELLA

African Story

In a bright sunny village, the much-loved Chief was very weak and dying a slow death. He lay on his mat surrounded by healing shamans who danced and sang. They made offerings and beat drums, but none of this did any good at all. No one could save him.

Young Mella, his child, was deep in distress for love of her father. Fingering the crescent moon amulet that she wore around her neck, she wandered into the forest by night, calling on the Moon Goddess, Bomo Rambi. The Goddess came to Mella who told her about her father. The Goddess spoke directly.

'You must go to the Python Healer. You must go to the Python Healer.'

Mella was terrified. Others had visited his cave and the few who returned had brought tales of horror about what they had seen there. Mella tried to put Bomo Rambi's words out of her mind, but try as she would to forget, she knew what she must do.

For four days and four nights she travelled through ferns and rocks and wooded mountains, and she crossed streams, all the while bravely singing songs to keep her heart true. The birds and creatures sang with her in support, but on the fourth day everything fell silent. A spiral on the rock marked the home of the Python Healer. She had arrived.

Struggling to find her voice and speak, Mella remembered why she had come.

'I am Mella sent by Bomu Rambi. For many moons my father lies sick. Will you help me?'

A pair of dark eyes peered from the cave and a voice as frightening as can be imagined spoke.

'A girl has come to my cave? Do you not know I could crush and strangle you, even as you stand before me?'

In terror, Mella told the Python Healer that her fear was great, but above all she loved her father and the love for him was stronger than her terror, and therefore he must listen to her.

'If your love is so great,' he said, 'turn your back and allow me to slither and twine myself around you!'

Gathering all the love in her heart, Mella turned her back. He twisted himself around her once, twice and three times. Her love for her father was so great she let him cover her, head to foot, so that she could not be seen. He instructed her to carry him and walk the four long days and nights back to the village. And despite her fear she did this.

Arriving back at the village, the people raised their spears to attack, but Mella shouted, 'Stop! It is I, Mella. I bring healing for our father.'

And they both passed into village to the mat of the dying Chief. From his neck the Python Healer took a pouch of healing bark and a deer horn of muchonga oil. He told Mella to set fire to the bark-oil and let incense rise all around. As she did this, the Python Healer spoke out the holy chants over the dying man.

It was like magic. The Chief slowly began to wake and sit up, and then he came to his feet, and finally he walked. Everyone could see he was healed and there was a feast and joyful celebration. The Python Healer told Mella she must now take him home. He twined around her exhausted body and they set out. Four days and four nights.

When they arrived, he asked her to enter his cave where there were the most amazing jewels and riches. The Python Healer told Mella to pick a gift from him to mark her heart of courage. Mella asked the Python Healer to choose and he found an amulet, a crescent moon, which, strange as it may seem, fitted perfectly with the one she always wore and which had been hers from birth.

For many years, the Chief lived bountifully, but eventually it was his time and he died peacefully. After a suitable mourning, Mella became Queen. Her first act was to carve a statue as an exact likeness to the Python Healer. She had it placed in a prominent position in the village so that all would remember the crescent moon of Bomo Rambi and the care she has for those who live with love and a heart of courage for healing.

THE MYSTERIES OF ORPHEUS
Greek Myth

Once there lived Orpheus whose gift was music. When he sang and played, even the plants would turn in recognition, because the melody he made lived also somewhere within them.

For many years Orpheus practised in the service of his music. But there came the day when his heart asked for something more. Soon after this, he fell in love with Eurydice, a woman so beautiful that his soul felt that it had come home. They loved one another and marriage made them one. The wedding celebration outdid any before it.

It was just after the wedding that Eurydice was pursued by a man who appeared at first to be a simple shepherd. He made to embrace her, and, when escaping his touch, Eurydice stepped on a snake which bit her. When Orpheus found her, she was dead. Zeus, King of all the Gods, was moved by the suffering of Orpheus. They spoke together, and it was agreed that Orpheus could travel to the underworld, where he would seek Eurydice, to see if there were conditions by which she could return from that land.

Full of hope, Orpheus took up his songs again. He made his way to the cave which led deep down, by unknown ways, to the River Styx. Crossing the river, he soothed Cerberus, the three-headed gatekeeper dog, by singing to him and so winning his trust and gaining entrance to the Land of the Dead. Orpheus descended and, at each step, the shades of the dead were touched by his song of life. As they listened, they could feel again and recapture the life flow which once had been their birth right. Eventually, Orpheus reached the dark courts of King Hades and his Queen Persephone, where he played and sang with a whole heart, begging that his loved one be returned. It was granted that Orpheus could have his Eurydice if he led her back to the light. She would follow and he must trust this, without seeing or looking back. This was the condition.

So it was, they set off on their journey of return. Orpheus sang and again the spirits were soothed by his music. Just at the transition point, at the place where darkness surrenders to light, Orpheus doubted Eurydice. Was she with him as had been promised? He turned to be reassured by the face of his beloved, but as he did so, she let out a gasp and vanished back to the dark. That was the end of it. It was finished.

Distraught, failed and lost, Orpheus had nowhere to rest. Love had gone, but the music would not leave him. He wandered away from the dwellings of humankind, into the forest, to live by a river where he played songs of utmost grief.

There are many endings to this story. Some say that the wine women of Thrace, worshippers of Dionysius, found him there and tore him to pieces because he would have none of their passion. They cut off his head and gave it to the river, which carried it to the Island of Lesbos, where his songs can still be heard. Others say that his body was buried in the earth, and that a skylark eternally sang over it. Some believe that the Gods were so moved by his sadness that they took his lyre and cast it to the stars where it became a constellation for all to see and remember.

And it is also said that Orpheus became a priest and taught the mysteries of his journey. They say he sings as an oracle for souls needing music to accompany them into the ways of death, when they most need an unexpected gift from the darkness.

THE MYTH OF ER

Greece, Plato

Will you listen to my tale of a great hero named Er, who was slain in battle and after twelve days returned to life to tell people what he had seen? This story is for you and it may be about you.

After the battle, the soul of Er left his body and journeyed with a crowd of souls, travelling to a mysterious meadow, in which there were two passages. One led back down through the earth, while the other opened up high into the heavens. In-between sat Judges who directed the souls of the just upwards by the heavenly road, and the souls of evildoers downwards towards the earth, by the lower road. The Judges told Er that he was to be their messenger and report what he witnessed to humankind so that they would know. And Er agreed to write it down.

Watching, Er saw souls endlessly coming and going, returning from both directions to pass before the Judges. Some were dusty and worn, others clean and bright. Those who knew each other greeted and embraced. The just were full of joyous stories, while the evildoers mourned what they had endured for so long. They all camped out as if at a festival, sharing songs and stories of their journey above or below. There in that meadow-place they tarried for seven days.

On the eighth day, they journeyed on to a pillar of rainbow light, which stretched upwards and downwards, piercing the heaven and the earth. It was explained to Er that this was the axis which holds the heavens and earth in place. If he looked, he would see that at its centre sat Necessity, turning a spindle on her lap which rotated eight circles of whirling colour. Each colour circle had its own Siren who sang one single note which belonged to her. The eight voices of the Sirens, when heard together, made up the harmony music of the spheres. Underneath the throne of Necessity sat her three daughters: Lachesis who sings of the past, Clotho who sings of the present and Atropos who sings of the future. It took Er time to understand this. He had to be shown several times to grasp what was being explained to him and how to write it down.

As Er watched, an Interpreter came forward. He brought lots from the lap of Necessity and scattered them, in this way deciding the order in which the souls would choose their next life. Then he spread out the life choices. He told them, 'The time has come for you to make your decision. Be warned! Choose wisely! For the decision you make is in your hands alone. It cannot be revoked.' Some souls took his warning and chose carefully, but others were rash and chose what they thought would be a rich or easy life. They say that Odysseus was left until the end and found an insignificant life, rejected by others, but which he was glad to take, so that he could rest after all his previous adventures.

When each had chosen their life, the souls returned to Lachesis, who gave each a daemon or genius, to be the protector and fulfiller of the life choice. Clotho then confirmed the union, by spinning the life choice and the daemon into a single thread, on her spindle. And Atropos took this thread and plaited it so that it could never be snapped or broken. When this was done, each soul and daemon passed by Necessity and made homage, bowing down before her.

Then the souls were tired, but they moved on in scorching heat, across the plain of Leithe, until they arrived at the River of Unmindfulness where they drank deeply, not knowing that, by drinking, all that had gone before would be forgotten. There they fell asleep.

In the middle of the night, a great storm arose and the Earth quaked. The souls were awoken and thrown upwards like shooting stars, scattering here and there, each to be born on Earth, to the very place and time where they could each fulfil their destiny.

Er was prevented from drinking the water and so was able to remember it. He took what he had written and returned to the people to let them know all the things he had seen.

PRINCE RING

German Fairytale, Grimm

Once, a Prince named Ring was hunting in a wood when he saw a deer with a golden ring in her horns. When he tried to follow her, she disappeared into a thick mist, no longer to be seen. Coming into a clearing, he found an old woman hunched over a barrel. She told him a ring was inside, and when he leaned over, she shoved him in, sealed the barrel and sent it out to sea.

After a time, the barrel arrived on a shore where an old Giant found and released Ring and took him home to meet his Giant Wife. The Giants were kind. They told Ring that he could go anywhere in their home, except the kitchen. However, Ring heard a voice from the kitchen calling, 'Choose me. Choose me,' and he was very curious.

One day, the Giants told Ring that it was time for them to leave, and that Ring could have anything he wished to take with him on his journey. Ring asked for what was in the kitchen. The Giants were not happy, but because they had promised Ring anything he asked for, they went to the kitchen with him and released a dog called Snati-Snati. The dog was overjoyed to be with Ring, and the two decided to travel on together.

Ring and Snati-Snati found their way to a neighbouring land and to the palace of a King, who provided hospitality for Ring. The chief minister, Rauder, was jealous of the royal newcomer and advised the King to set up a challenge. Ring and Rauder must compete to see who could cut down most trees in the forest. Snati-Snati begged Ring for an axe and chopped down many more trees than Rauder. So Ring won! A second challenge was set. Ring was told to enter a field of wild bulls and remove their skin and horns and bring these to the King. Ring was daunted by the task, but, helped by Snati-Snati who ferociously killed the bulls, he accomplished the task and the King praised him. Rauder, still not satisfied, demanded that the King challenge Ring to retrieve golden treasure, stolen by a grotesque witch giantess, who lived high in the mountains with her family. Ring and Snati-Snati took a bag of salt to the giant's home and waited till they slept. Then they emptied the salt into the food, and when the giants became desperate for water and rushed from the cave to drink, Ring and Snati-Snati retrieved the gold and returned it to the

King. The King was delighted and gave Prince Ring the hand of his daughter in marriage.

On the evening before the wedding, Snati-Snati insisted on sleeping in Ring's bed. He also commanded Ring to sleep on the floor. During the night, Rauder, still consumed with jealousy, stole into Ring's room, crept towards the bed and raised a knife to kill the Prince. But Snati-Snati was ready. He bit off Rauder's right hand. The castle awoke to screams of Rauder who tried to hide his handless arm. But the King saw clearly for the first time and banished Rauder from the land for ever.

That night, Snati-Snati slept at the foot of Ring's bed, and because he did this, his form changed from dog into another Prince. This Prince also bore the name of Ring. He had long been under the enchantment of a wicked witch, but now he was released. The two Princes vowed they would never separate and would always live in friendship together.

PSYCHE AND EROS
Greek Myth

There once was a King who had three daughters. The youngest, Psyche, was very beautiful. Her loveliness was so great that she outshone the Goddess Aphrodite who became deeply jealous and wanted rid of her. Aphrodite instructed her son Eros to fire one of his love arrows into the heart of a monster so that Psyche would marry the fiend and would no longer be wooed and adored by all men. However, the plan went awry, for Eros pricked himself on his own arrow and Psyche, on seeing him, loved him.

Worried about the future of his youngest daughter, the King consulted the Oracle asking how a husband might be found. He did not know that Aphrodite had instructed the Oracle to say that Psyche must be dressed as a bride and taken to a high crag outside the city and left there. Followed by a long procession of wailing and tears, Psyche was bound and taken and abandoned to the coming of her fate.

However, the West Wind who had been watching took pity on her. He lifted her away to a great palace where she was lovingly attended. She could hear voices and feel presence, but never once did she see the hands that served her. At night a prince came to her bed and loved her tenderly, but she never saw his face. All was well as long as she never demanded to see.

In time Psyche's sisters came to visit. They saw her happiness and the richness of her palace and were consumed with envy. They questioned, was her lover blighted, or was he a monster, or maybe even an old man? She should light a lamp and look with her own eyes, and a knife close by, so that if her beloved was repulsive, she could kill him.

Persuaded, Psyche lit an oil lamp and looked. She saw that it was none other than Eros who lay beside her. Her hand trembled and a drop of oil fell from the lamp on to his wings. He awoke, and because love dies when trust is broken, he spread his great wings and flew from her. Psyche was distraught at what she had done. She ran to the river to throw herself in, but the God Pan spoke to her sternly, telling her she must not give up but instead search endlessly for Eros. And, saved from her death, she set out.

Meanwhile, a seagull had told Aphrodite that Psyche was with child through Eros. Demented at the idea of being a grandmother, she sent her servant 'Old Habit' to bring Psyche to her. As soon as the girl arrived, Aphrodite had her beaten and then locked her into to a large room filled with beans and peas. She told Psyche to separate these into two piles by morning or she would die. Wearily, Psyche tried, but the task was too much. Had it not been for an army of ants who accomplished the work by dawn, it would not have been possible.

But Aphrodite was not satisfied. She demanded that Psyche collect golden fleece from a fierce flock of rams in a field nearby. This was impossible as the rams attacked anyone coming close. Despairing, Psyche noticed that the bullrushes were speaking to her. They told her to wait until evening when the rams would sleep, for then she could gather the fleece from the bramble thorns growing around the field. So Psyche waited and gathered the golden fleece by morning.

Still, the Goddess was not finished. She insisted that Psyche fetch water from a dragon-filled river. This time Psyche was helped by an eagle who flew her safely on his back, so that she could collect the water and no dragon could reach her.

Aphrodite set one last task. She ordered Psyche to travel to Hades to bring back a beauty lotion which belonged to Persephone, Queen of the Dead, and she must on no account look at it. She told Psyche that if anyone asked her for help, she must ignore them.

Now this warning was needed. Kind-hearted Psyche was approached three times. An old man on a donkey tried to delay her, asking her to rescue him from the darkness of the underworld. But she passed on. When crossing the great river, she heard someone calling her name from the water. A man she knew there was drowning. But she passed on. And then three old women beseeched her to stop and listen to their woes. But Psyche moved away from them and passed right on.

She found the box with its potion within but, oh, it tempted her. Just one look, she thought as she lifted the lid. And when she saw, Psyche fell deathlike to the ground. It was there that Eros found her a little later and he could do nothing to wake her.

Eros flew to the Gods of Olympus, begging them to give Psyche immortality so she could be his. Eventually, this was agreed. Hermes was sent to bring her to Olympus where she was welcomed. A cup of ambrosia was drunk by all the Gods, and Psyche was given wings so that she could fly with Eros in their eternal union of love. Even Aphrodite was satisfied, for now men would look again to her beauty and worship as was right. And there was no one to surpass her.

THE QUEEN BEE

German Fairytale, Grimm

A King had three sons. When they grew up, the two eldest went in search of adventure. They fell into dissolute ways and never came home. Then the youngest son, who was known as Simpleton, went in search of his brothers. When he found them, they jeered at him for his simple ways, telling him that he would never get on in the world.

As the three were walking together, they came to an anthill. The two older brothers wanted to kick it open, to see the little ants rush about in terror and carry their eggs away. But Simpleton stopped them, insisting that they leave the creatures in peace.

Then they came to a lake with ducks swimming on it. The older brothers wanted to catch two of the ducks and roast them. But Simpleton stopped them, saying, 'I will not let you kill them. Leave them in peace.'

Further on they came to a bee's nest in a tree. The two older brothers wanted to make a fire under the tree and smoke the bees out so that they could take the honey. Again, Simpleton stopped them, saying, 'I will not let you burn the bees!'

The three brothers went on their way. After a while they came to a strange, silent castle. There were stone horses in the stable and stone people in the yard. At length they came to a door with three locks. In the middle of the door was a little pane through which they could see into a room where a small, grey man was seated at a table. They had to call him three times before he took any notice. He didn't speak but opened the door and led them to a room where a table was spread with good food.

After they had eaten, he led the way to three bedrooms and they all slept soundly. Next morning the little man led the eldest brother to a stone table on which were inscribed three tasks. He explained that if these tasks were carried out successfully, the castle would be freed from an enchantment. The first task was to find the princess's pearls, a thousand in number, which were under the moss in the nearby forest. If a single pearl was missing, the seeker would be turned to stone.

The eldest brother went to the forest and searched in the moss all day, but at the end of the day he had only found a hundred pearls. He was turned to stone.

On the second day, the second brother searched for the pearls, but at the end of the day he had found only two hundred. He, too, was turned to stone.

When Simpleton tried to find the pearls, he was so slow and found so few that he quickly realised his situation was hopeless, so he sat on a stone and wept. While he was sitting there, the King of the ants whose life he had saved came to his rescue with five thousand ants. Simpleton could see the earth and moss moving all around him and it was not long before the little creatures had gathered all the thousand pearls and laid them in front of him in a heap. So the first task was accomplished.

The second task was to find the key to the bedchamber of the King's daughters, which had been thrown in a nearby lake. Simpleton looked at the lake and again he despaired, but the ducks he had saved dived down and brought him the key.

The third task looked even harder than the other two. He was to enter the bedroom where three princesses were sleeping and identify the youngest and dearest princess. But they all looked exactly alike. The only difference between them was that, just before they fell asleep, each had tasted a different sweet. The eldest had eaten a piece of sugar; the second, a spoonful of syrup; and the youngest had eaten some honey. As Simpleton was looking from one princess to the other, the Queen of the bees, whom Simpleton had protected from the threat of fire, came buzzing through the window. Delicately, she tasted the lips of the three princesses and stayed on the mouth which had eaten honey.

So the King's youngest son was led by the Queen Bee to the youngest and dearest princess, the one with honey on her lips. In accomplishing the three tasks, Simpleton broke the enchantment which had turned all the people and animals in the castle to stone. The three princesses woke up and so did the King and Queen. Even Simpleton's older brothers came back to life and they married the other two princesses.

RAPUNZEL

German Fairytale, Grimm

Once upon a time, a man and a woman longed for a child. They were childless for many years, but then the woman became pregnant and they realised that their wish was to be granted. The window of their house looked out on a garden where their neighbour grew the most beautiful flowers and the most mouth-watering vegetables. The garden was surrounded by a high wall and belonged to a green-fingered witch who was feared throughout the neighbourhood.

One day the woman was sitting by the window, looking out at the garden, when she noticed a bed planted with the greenest, most delicious rapunzel, which is a special kind of lettuce. Every day she looked out and the rapunzel grew more appetising. She longed to eat some. She knew there was no way to get it, but she grew pale with longing until her husband asked her what was the matter. 'Oh,' she said, 'if I don't get to eat some of that lettuce that grows behind our house, I think I will die!' The man made up his mind to get some of that rapunzel for her, come what may. As soon as it was dark, he climbed into the garden and grabbed a handful. His wife made it into a salad which she ate greedily. Next day she was desperate for more and again her husband climbed the wall into the witch's garden. When he found the witch standing in front of him, he explained about his pregnant wife and the witch told him he could take some rapunzel on condition that they gave her the child they were expecting.

And so it was. The woman gave birth to a baby girl and a few days later the witch was on their doorstep to collect her. She called the girl Rapunzel and raised her as though she were her own daughter.

When Rapunzel was twelve years old, the witch took her into the forest and put her in a tower with no door and only one window, at the very top, telling her this was where she must live from now on. The witch, whom the girl believed to be her mother, promised to come with provisions every day and look after all her needs. She would call out, 'Rapunzel, Rapunzel, let down your hair!' When she heard this, the girl, who had very long, golden hair, must unfasten her braids and let her hair down to the ground below so that the witch could climb up to the high window.

Rapunzel lived quietly in her tower for some time, weaving and spinning and singing to herself with a sweet voice. One day the King's son was riding through the forest and heard her singing. He was charmed by the sound and rode towards it, finding himself outside a tower with no door. Riding on, he was haunted by the memory of her song. He came back to the tower many times and stood there, listening. One day he saw the witch approaching the tower and heard her call out, 'Rapunzel, Rapunzel, let down your hair!' And he watched her climb up.

When the witch had gone, the Prince thought he would try his luck. He stood at the bottom of the tower and called, 'Rapunzel! Rapunzel! Let down your hair!' The hair cascaded from the window and he climbed up. When Rapunzel saw him, she was terrified. She had never seen a man before. But he talked to her kindly and gently and soon overcame her fear. She began to enjoy his company.

At last the Prince told her he loved her and asked her to come away with him. She replied that she could not leave the tower without his help. But if he would bring a skein of silk every time he visited her, she would weave a silk ladder, and when the ladder was long enough she would be able to climb down and ride away with him.

So he visited her every evening, while the old woman came during the day. The old witch noticed nothing unusual. But one evening Rapunzel innocently asked her, 'How is it, mother, that you are so much heavier for me to pull up than the King's son?'

The old woman was filled with rage. She scolded Rapunzel for deceiving her, seized a pair of scissors and cut off her long golden hair. Then she dragged the girl off to a desert place and shut her away in a hut where she wept tears of misery.

That evening when the young Prince called out, 'Rapunzel, Rapunzel, let down your hair,' and climbed up to the window of the tower, he discovered Rapunzel's golden hair on a hook that the witch had hung it from and the witch herself was there, waiting for him. She told him in a great rage that his bird had flown and the cat had got her. In despair, the Prince jumped from the window of the tower and fell on his face among the thorns below, which tore at his eyes and made him blind.

He did not return to his father's palace, but groped his way out of the forest and wandered through the world, grieving over his loss. After seven years he came to a hut in the desert and heard a woman singing inside. The sound was strangely familiar. He had come to the hut where Rapunzel was living in poverty with their twin children, a boy and a girl. Rapunzel recognised him and fell on his neck, weeping. As her soon as her tears touched his eyes, he found he could see again.

Then the Prince led Rapunzel and their two children back to his kingdom where they were welcomed with joy and lived in great happiness.

THE SACRED GIFT OF SONG,
──DANCE AND FESTIVITY──
Inuit Legend

Once upon a time, the Mother of the Earth World had become tired. She looked down over her people and could see no joy mirrored in them. Beat by beat, her heart became slower and fainter. She had become tired and hopeless.

She sent out to the world. She needed someone to make the journey to visit her, but no one arrived. When she was at her most exhausted, she called to her son, Eagle Man, begging for his help. After time, he returned with a youthful man, the youngest of three sons. He was the only one who had agreed to make the journey to her, although his two brothers had each been invited.

Great Mother said to the man, 'My heart is almost gone. I need you to call a great celebration on the Earth. There must be singing and dancing, music and playing. Creatures must celebrate. Will you do this?' She told him how to build a celebration hut and how to teach beings to dance. She told him how to make a feast and how to sing. For a whole night there should be dance, and song, and the making of music. Every person must find their joy song, every person create their dance.

So the young man returned to his parents, who welcomed him back for they had sorely missed him. They helped him build the celebration hut and learned how to sing. Soon all was ready for the celebration. People and creatures all arrived. They feasted, they danced, they sang, and the Earth was a celebration all night long. And then they quietly slept the remainder of the night and dreamed the dream they most needed to follow.

When the early dawn arose, a sound was heard coming from above. It was the strong beat of the Mother's heart, echoing the joy on earth. All was well again.

THE SEAL WOMAN
Scotland

Many years ago a young farmer man lived on a small island off the west coast of Scotland. He was born there and both his parents were dead, so he had the island to himself, working the farm and living in the house they left him. He loved to wander along the shore and watch the wild creatures.

Some days he went across the water to sell his produce, and people in the market would tease him, saying, 'What are you up to, living alone on that island? Isn't it time you found yourself a wife?' But he would laugh and answer back, 'I'm better off on my own. Think of Adam. Who got him turned out of Paradise?'

One evening, when the tide was out, he went for a stroll on the island and came to a cave. He was surprised to hear the sound of music. Looking through a hole in the rock, he saw some young people dancing. They were all naked, with pale skins and beautiful faces. Outside the cave, close to the water, was a pile of sealskins. The young man thought, 'One of those would make a good warm coat for the winter.' He picked himself a fine, silky skin and walked home with it.

Next morning the sealskin was still wet, so he put it away over the lintel of the barn door. Then, remembering the young people he had seen dancing in the cave, he decided to go back and see if they were still there. As he approached the cave, he heard someone crying. He discovered a young woman seated on a rock, weeping bitterly. For the first time in his life, the young man who had scorned women recognised that here was someone he could care about.

The woman looked at him with her beautiful brown eyes and asked if he would help her to find her sealskin, as without it she could never return to her home or see her people again. Knowing stories about the seal people, he recognised who she was. But how could he bear to return the sealskin and lose her?

He said nothing, just took her in his arms and offered to look after her, taking her back to the farm and giving her bread, milk and a bed to lie on. The young man was kind and gentle and the seal woman learnt to love him. At last they were married and she gave birth to four beautiful children, two boys and two girls. She loved her children and looked after them well, but there were days when she would wander by the shore and look out over the waves, singing strange and beautiful songs that brought tears to the eyes of all who heard them.

The years passed and one day, when the farmer was out working in his fields and the boys were playing on the beach, the two girls went to play in the barn and found a strange, silky skin tucked over the lintel. They pulled it down and took it into the house to show to their mother, asking her what it was.

When she saw it, the seal woman reached for the skin and held it against her face, singing quietly to herself. She took her children in her arms, held them close for a few moments and then ran out of the house, down to the edge of the sea. Wrapping the skin around herself, she plunged into the waves and disappeared from view.

The farmer returned from his fields that evening to find his children huddled by an empty hearth. When they told him what had happened, he said, 'My poor children, I don't think we'll be seeing your mother in this house ever again.' He lit the fire and cooked their supper that night and every night that followed. He never married again, for no woman ever stirred his heart as the seal woman had. And she did not return.

But at times when the children were playing on the beach near their home, a seal would swim in near the shore and watch them with its big brown eyes. It never came any closer, but the sight of it always comforted them.

THE SNOW QUEEN

Denmark, Hans Christian Anderson

An evil goblin made a magic mirror that had the power to distort beauty into ugliness. He took the mirror into the heavens hoping to fool the angels, but it slipped, shattering into billions of splinters, which were blown into people's hearts and eyes, and caused them to see only the bad in themselves and in other people.

About this time, Kay and Gerda lived in the high garrets of two buildings with adjoining roofs. They shared a window-box garden where they grew roses, and they loved each other dearly as playmates, until a mirror fragment fell into Kay's heart. He completely changed and became cruel and hard. He destroyed the window box and became derisive of Gerda. The only thing that he loved was the snow that came with winter.

One day a sleigh came into the town on which sat the Snow Queen wearing white fur and as cold as ice. To steal a fast ride, Kay attached his little sledge to the back of her sleigh. She spied Kay and took him up beside her, kissing him twice, once to numb him from feeling her ice, and the second time to make him forget about Gerda and his family. She took him to her palace near the North Pole where he thought himself content with her.

Gerda was heartbroken when Kay disappeared. She questioned everyone, even the river who sent her to a kind old witch woman, who took Gerda into her enchanted garden where it was always summer. The witch wanted to keep Gerda, so she hid all the roses in the garden and brushed Gerda's hair so she forgot everything. One day Gerda found a rose which the witch had failed to hide and she remembered Kay. She tore herself from the softness of the garden and its eternal summer. Outside, a raven spoke to her. He told her that he had seen a boy just like Kay, married to a princess who lived very close by. Gerda made her way there, but when she saw the prince, it was not Kay. Gerda told the prince and princess her story and they wanted to help her. They gave her warm clothes and a beautiful coach, full of good things to eat on the journey.

But robbers on the hunt for gold attacked Gerda. They almost killed her, but a little girl robber wanted Gerda for her friend, so she stayed with the robbers for some time. One night the wood pigeons in the roof told Gerda that they had seen Kay at the North Pole. The robber girl said that she would help Gerda by giving her a reindeer who knew the way to Lapland. Gratefully, Gerda and the reindeer set off. On the journey they stopped at the home of a Lapp woman, and then, moving even further northwards, they came to the home of a Finn woman who told Gerda about the splinter of glass in Kay's heart. She assured Gerda that she had love enough to shift it.

Gerda arrived. She saw Kay, blue with cold, for the Snow Queen had turned his heart to ice. He sat playing with shafts of ice, for the Snow Queen had said if he could use them to spell out the word ETERNITY, he could go home. But he could not do it. It was only when Gerda's warm tears ran down his face, on to his chest, that his ice-heart melted and he could see her. The tears dislodged the splinter from his eye, and he danced for joy with Gerda, so that the ice shafts magically joined the dance and fell to ground in the form of the word that was so greatly needed. ETERNITY.

Kay and Gerda were free to leave the Snow Queen's domain, so they made their way home. When they arrived there, everything was the same, but they had changed, for they were almost grown up. It was no longer winter and the cold had gone. The summer had come, and it would stay, for a very long time.

THE STAR WOMAN
Bushmen, South Africa

Once, in the days of the early race, there was a man who captured a superb herd of cattle, all stippled in black and white. He loved them very much. Every day he took them out to graze, and brought them home in the evenings, put them in his thorn shelter and milked them in the morning. One morning, he found that they had already been milked; their udders, which had been sleek the night before, were wrinkled and dry. He thought, 'Well, this is very extraordinary. I couldn't have looked after them very well yesterday,' and he took them to better grazing. But again the next morning he found that they had been milked. That night, bringing them back after a good feed, he sat up to watch. About midnight, he saw a cord come down from the stars, and down this cord, hand over hand, came young women of the people of the stars. He saw them with calabashes and baskets, whispering among themselves, creep into the shelter and start to milk his cattle. He took up his stick and he ran for them. Immediately, they scattered and, running for the cord, they went up as fast as they could.

He managed to catch one of them by the leg and pull her back. She was the loveliest of them all and he married her. Their life would have been happy but for one thing. She had with her, when he caught her, a tightly woven basket with a lid fitted tightly into its neck. She said to him, 'There is only one thing I ask of you and that is that you will never look into this basket without my permission.' He promised. Every day she went out to cultivate the fields as women do and he went to look after the cattle and to hunt. This went on for some months, but gradually the sight of this basket in the corner began to annoy him. One day, coming back for a drink of water in the middle of the day, when his wife was away in the fields, he saw the basket standing there and he said, 'Well, really, this is too much. I'm going to have to look into it.' He pulled up the lid of the basket, looked inside and began to laugh. In the evening his wife came back and after one look at him she knew what had happened. She said, 'You've looked in the basket.' He said, 'Yes, I have,' and then added, 'You silly, silly woman. The basket is empty.' She said, 'You saw nothing in the basket?' 'No, nothing.' Thereupon, looking very sad, she turned her back on him and vanished into the sunset.

STONE SOUP

European Folk Tale

A tramp had been on the road for some days and towards evening he came to a village. Being hungry, he knocked on a few doors asking for food. The people in the village were mean and nobody gave him anything. At last he paused by a little bridge and looked down at the stream below, wondering what he could do to get a meal. He caught sight of a large, well-rounded stone at the water's edge and had an idea. Picking up the stone, he dried it carefully, wrapped it in a piece of bright silk and put it in his pocket. Then he walked to the middle of the village and knocked on the door of a house.

An old woman opened the door and asked, not too politely, what he wanted. He replied that he wasn't asking for anything. On the contrary, he had come to offer her a taste of his wonderful stone soup. All he needed was the loan of a saucepan and a little water and he would prepare the most delicious soup for her.

The old woman liked the idea of someone cooking her evening meal and she was curious to taste the soup. She produced a pan and the man filled it with water, placing it on the kitchen stove. Then he unwrapped the stone and carefully put it in the water. Soon steam was rising from the pot. The tramp asked for a spoon, gave the pot a stir and said, 'I don't suppose you have an onion, do you? It will taste even better if we put in an onion.'

'Well, yes, I do,' said the old woman. She was getting excited at the prospect of supper. She brought two onions which he peeled and put into the pan. Then he asked if she had any carrots.

The old woman didn't have any carrots, but she didn't want to spoil the soup so she said, 'Just wait a minute and I'll get some.' She hurried next door to beg some carrots from her neighbour, telling her about the wonderful stone soup her visitor was making. The neighbour became curious and asked if she could come and watch the cooking.

When they got back to her house, the tramp was still stirring the pot. He peeled the carrots, added them to the mixture and went on stirring. Then he said, 'It would be even better if we put in a few cabbage leaves!'

More neighbours were drawn in and more vegetables added to the pot, parsnips and potatoes and salt and herbs, and even a few chicken bones. Eventually, the soup was ready. All agreed that it was the best soup they had ever tasted.

The neighbours went home, the bowls were washed up. Then the tramp washed his stone, dried it very carefully and wrapped it in the piece of bright silk. As he was about to tuck it into his pocket, the old woman asked if he would consider selling it.

THE STORY BAG
Korean Folk Tale

Once upon a time, there was a boy who loved to hear stories more than anything. However, when his friends asked him to tell them, he relentlessly refused. So the spirits of the stories had nowhere to go, and they were crammed into a leather bag which hung on a nail in the boy's bedroom. Each time a new story was told, the story spirit was added and the bag grew tighter and tighter and there was no room. In time, sadly, the boy's parents died. Eventually, a servant took on the job of telling him tales, but he always refused to share them.

After a while, the boy grew up and his rich uncle found him a wife. On the day of the wedding, whilst the young man was bathing, the servant overheard the spirits muttering in the bag.

One said, 'Within my story is a poisoned well. Today, as he travels, I shall become that well and lure him to drink from me.'

A second said, 'If that does not work, I hold a field of lush, red strawberries. I will appear to him, and when he eats I will choke him to death on the first taste.'

The third said, 'If you are not successful, I contain a red hot poker. My plan is to bury myself in the rice sack that acts as a step from his carriage. When he steps out, I will scorch all the life out of him!'

And a fourth quiet little story spirit said, 'I am about a snake with venom. I will place myself nightwards, at the foot of his wedding bed, and wait for him there.'

The servant tried to tell the young man what he had heard, but he would not listen. So the servant begged permission to lead the carriage horse on the journey to the wedding, and this favour was agreed.

The young man set out, and as he travelled, he saw a well from which he longed to drink. But the servant refused to stop! Soon the young man smelled strawberries and craved them, but the servant drove the horse on! Later, as the young man stepped from the carriage, the servant hurled himself upon his master, knocking him sideways before he reached the rice sack! The young man was furious! He strongly reprimanded the servant for his mean behaviour and sent him to the lowest seat at the feast.

Just before midnight, when the nuptial bed was ready, into that most intimate moment burst the servant. He whipped off the bed clothes, revealed the snake and removed it. At last he was allowed to explain all that had gone on before.

From that day on, the man knew he could no longer trap stories in a bag and keep them as if hidden. He became responsible for releasing all kinds of stories and giving them to others who valued them. And the spirits of the stories became free and available for everyone, as they wanted to be.

THE TENGU

Japan

A long time ago there lived in Japan a monstrous firebird known as the Tengu. One day it pounced on a young water dragon that lived in the garden of a Buddhist monastery. The dragon was too small to fight the Tengu, but hung helplessly in the firebird's talons. The Tengu flew with the young water dragon to a desert country and dropped it into a cleft in a rock, leaving it there to die. Then it flapped its great wings and flew straight back to the monks' garden.

A monk had been drawing water from the well and was walking round the garden, pitcher in hand, searching for the little water dragon. When the Tengu's shadow fell on the monk, he looked up and realised immediately what had happened. The monk shook his fist at the firebird.

The Tengu, because it is irresistibly attracted to anger in any form, swooped down and carried off the angry monk. It dropped him into the same cleft of dry rock where the water dragon lay broken and half dead. The monk spread out his sleeves as he fell from the Tengu's talons and floated gently down to the cleft in the rock. Most of the water in his pitcher had spilled, but there was just a little left. He poured this with his blessings on the little water dragon's head. At the first touch of pure water, the water dragon began to grow. It swelled and swelled like a storm cloud, lashed its rainbow tail and broke the rocks apart. The monk climbed on the back of the water dragon and together they flew back to the garden.

A THORN IN THE KING'S FOOT
Scotland, the Travelling People

Many years ago, there was a powerful king who took half of what his people earned in taxes. He was proud of his wealth and didn't care that his people were poor and unhappy. He spent most of his time hunting and he neglected his Queen, not noticing that she was lonely. She longed for a child, but the years went by and still she had no child to keep her company.

One day, when the King was boasting of their riches, the Queen turned to him and said, 'Husband, all the riches in the world will never make me happy.' The king was astonished and distressed because, in his way, he loved his Queen. He asked what he could do and she said that the only thing she wanted was a child.

The King listened, for the first time in his life, to someone else's wish. He began to spend more time with her and the Queen conceived. She gave birth to a baby boy with golden hair and blue eyes and she loved him dearly, but he was a hunchback.

When the King saw the hump on his back, he cast the baby aside, saying, 'This is no child of mine!' The baby prince grew into a happy child and all who knew him loved him. But the King avoided him. He never took him out to meet the people, though they knew there was a baby prince. The King knew this could not go on.

One day he sent for two of his huntsmen and ordered them to take the child into the forest, kill him and bring back the proof. They took the child during the night and rode with him to a distant part of the forest. All the time the little boy smiled at them in his trusting way. They couldn't bring themselves to harm him, so they left him under a tree, wrapped in a small blanket. Then they killed a young deer to take its heart back to the king.

The baby slept soundly. Waking in the early morning, he just lay under the tree, quietly listening to the noises of the forest. An old woman who lived in the forest found him there as she was gathering sticks for her fire. She loved him on sight and made up her mind to take care of him.

This old woman lived alone in the forest on her own because of a disease that created ugly blemishes on her face, a disease known as the King's evil which, it was said, could be cured by the touch of a King. So she hid herself away from other people, keeping hens and goats and growing vegetables. She enjoyed the freedom of the forest and hid her face behind a veil if ever she had to go into the town. The boy settled into a new life with her in the forest and never seemed to notice anything wrong with her face.

At court it was announced that the baby had died. The King ordered a small coffin and held a mock funeral, putting on a show of grief. But the Queen could not be comforted. She refused to eat, and when the King pleaded with her, all she could say was 'I don't want anything. I just want my baby.'

After a few days she died. Now the King was inconsolable, knowing in his heart that he had caused his Queen's death and that if he could have overcome his feelings about the child being a hunchback, his Queen would still be alive and happy. Years passed and nothing changed. The sad King no longer went hunting, but stayed grieving in his palace.

One day he thought that if he went out and talked with his people, that might bring him some comfort. He walked into the town, but when people saw his sad face, they just said, 'Sorry, your Majesty!' and walked on. They didn't stop and talk because they didn't love him.

Suddenly he caught sight of a woman in a veil. As she walked past him, he heard her say, 'On your way, Majesty, and a curse on you!' The King couldn't believe his ears. He asked, 'What did you say, woman?'

But she walked on without replying and the King felt something sharp go into his foot. As he walked on, it became very painful and by the time he got back to the Palace it was hurting so much that he retired to his bed and sent for his doctors. They bathed his foot and put on healing oils, but nothing helped the pain. The King became convinced that he had a thorn in his foot, but the doctors could not find anything. After a while a green shoot appeared, growing out of the King's big toe. It sprouted, grew branches and put on leaves. A small thorn tree was growing out of the King's foot and no one could do anything about it. The King just lay there in agony with his foot resting on the window ledge and a tree growing out of his big toe. People came from far and wide to offer remedies but no one could shift it. The only respite the King knew was when a cool wind blew out of the forest. Then, for a while, the pain would subside and he would get some rest.

Through the years of the King's suffering, his son was growing into a young man, looked after by the old woman in the forest. She called him 'Robin' because of his bright eyes when she found him under the tree. He called her Mother, remembering no other parent. She taught him how to grow food, look after the hens and goats and hunt in the forest. And she gave him wisdom by telling him stories. All that time she felt her face getting uglier with the disease, but the boy didn't seem to notice. He loved her because she was kind and he specially loved her voice, telling stories by the fire.

One evening the old woman told him a story she had never told before. She told him she was not his mother, that his real mother had been a Queen who loved him but died of grief after the King got rid of him.

By now Robin was a strong, good-looking young man, even with his hunched back. He remembered nothing but kindness and was shocked by the old woman's story. He said, 'What has this got to do with me? If the King didn't want me then as a son, he won't want me now.'

The old woman said, 'There is something else you need to know. Your father is suffering because of something I did to him. You are the only person who can help him. At the same time, you can help me to get a cure for the disease that makes my face so ugly.'

He protested that as far as he was concerned there was nothing wrong with her face. But she said she was tired of hiding away from the world and that the sores on her face were caused by the 'King's evil', which could only be cured by the touch of a king.

Then she told him what he could do to make her happy and at the same time rescue the King and make the whole country a happier place. She said, 'You must walk into the town, knock on the door of the Palace and tell them you have come to heal the King's foot. They will admit you because the King is in despair. Don't tell the King who you are. Just say that you can heal his foot, but first he must make two promises: that he will go with you to the forest and touch my face, and that he will leave you to rule over his kingdom for two hundred days and go to live among his people, disguised as a poor man.'

Robin protested that it wouldn't work, that he was not qualified to rule the country, but the woman insisted, 'You are qualified. You are a king's son. But don't tell him that until the two hundred days have passed.'

Robin went to the Palace, was taken to the King and found him with his foot out of the window, saying, 'It's impossible. No one can cure me.'

He assured the King that he could cure him, but on two conditions. He must come and heal the woman in the forest. And then he must let Robin rule the country for two hundred days while he went among his people, disguised as a poor man.

The King, being desperate, agreed and Robin gently eased the thorn tree out of the King's foot and dropped it from the window to the ground below. Then he passed his hand over the foot. All the pain left it and he told the King to stand up.

The King stood, walked across the room and sent for two horses. They rode into the forest together and found the old woman. The King touched her face and the disease was healed, leaving her face lined with age but clear and beautiful. Then they rode back to the Palace and the King told his councillors that Robin was going to rule the country for a while. He put on some old and shabby clothes and walked out of the Palace.

As he walked along the road, the King felt a weight lift from his shoulders. He got work on a farm and was paid a small wage. Unknown to his people, he lived among them and, to his surprise, he enjoyed himself. With Robin in charge of the land, people began to notice changes. Taxes were lowered and they were no longer poor. The King, in his disguise, noticed that his people were happier. The two hundred days seemed to pass very quickly.

Returning to the Palace, the King said, 'Robin, you have done more than cure my foot. You have shown me how to be happy and how to rule my kingdom! Why don't you stay in the Palace and be my Prime Minister?'

Then Robin said, 'Father, you denied me once because I was a hunchback. If a hunchback was no good to you as a son, why would I be any good to you as a Prime Minister?'

The King begged his son's forgiveness and pleaded with him to stay, but he would not, insisting that his home was in the forest with the mother who had been kind to him. He said, 'If you want to see me any time, you will find me there.' And he walked away from the Palace.

THOUSANDFURS

German Fairytale, Grimm

There was a King whose wife had golden hair and was incomparably beautiful. They were happy together, but the Queen became ill. When she knew that she was dying, she told the King that if he ever wished to marry again, he must find a wife as beautiful as she was, with hair as golden as hers.

She died and the King could not be comforted. He had no wish to marry again. But as time passed, his councillors began to say that the country needed another Queen. Remembering her dying words, the King sent messengers across the land to search for a woman as beautiful as his late Queen. They searched and searched but found no one who could be compared with her.

The King had a daughter who was growing to womanhood. One day he caught sight of her walking past a window and noticed that she was as beautiful as her mother, with hair as golden. He fell completely in love and told his councillors that he was going to marry his daughter.

The councillors were shocked, protesting that it was forbidden for a father to marry his daughter, but his resolution could not be shaken. His daughter was even more shocked and did her best to change his mind, but she could not. At last, appearing to give in, she told him that before fulfilling his wish she must have three dresses, one as golden as the sun, one as silver as the moon and one as bright and shining as the stars. As well, she must have a cloak made of a thousand different furs and pelts, gathered from all the animals in his kingdom.

The King ordered the cleverest seamstresses to make the three dresses and the cleverest huntsmen to gather a thousand pieces of skin and fur for the cloak. It took time, but at last all was done and the King laid out his gifts before her, announcing that their wedding would take place the very next day.

The Princess saw that her situation was hopeless. That night, when everyone was asleep, she gathered up three little treasures: a golden ring, a golden spinning wheel and a golden reel. She packed the three dresses of the sun, moon and stars into a nutshell. Then she put on her cloak of a thousand furs, blackened her face and hands with soot and left her father's palace, walking into the forest and climbing into a hollow tree to sleep.

She slept past sunrise and into the next day. In the morning, another King was hunting in the forest and his dogs sniffed at the tree and ran around it, barking loudly. The King asked his huntsmen to look inside the tree and tell him what kind of beast was hiding there. They replied that that it was a beast such as they had never seen before, a beast with a thousand different furs. The King ordered them to catch it alive and bring it back to his palace.

When the huntsmen seized the girl, she told them she had been deserted by her parents and begged them to take her home with them. They took her back to the palace where she was told that she could live in a cupboard under the stairs and work in the kitchen, sweeping the hearth, carrying wood and water, and plucking chickens.

So the Princess lived and worked in the palace as a servant. One day a grand ball was held. Thousandfurs asked the cook if she could go upstairs and watch from behind a door. The cook allowed her to go, but only for half an hour. She washed her face and hands, took off her cloak of furs and put on the dress that was like the sun. When she walked into the ballroom, everyone stood aside and made way, as they would for a princess. The King had never seen anyone so beautiful and he danced with her. At the end of the dance she curtsied. The King turned away for a moment and she disappeared. No one could tell him where she had gone.

She had hurried back to her little den and turned herself back into Thousandfurs, returning to the kitchen. Now the cook wanted to go and watch the dancing, so he asked her to make the King's soup. She made some bread soup and into it she dropped her gold ring. When the ball was over, the King sent for his soup and found the ring at the bottom of the bowl. He sent for the cook and asked who had made the soup, saying that it tasted different from usual. When the cook confessed that it had been made by a hairy animal, the King sent for Thousandfurs. He asked her who she was and why she had put a gold ring in his soup. She denied all knowledge of the ring and said she was good for nothing but to have shoes thrown at her head.

Time passed and another ball was arranged. Again Thousandfurs got leave to watch the dancing and appeared in the silver dress, danced with the King and slipped away. Again she prepared his soup, putting the little golden spinning wheel in the bowl. And again, when the King sent for her, she stood before him as the hairy animal and denied all knowledge of the golden spinning wheel he had found in his soup.

When a third ball was held, Thousandfurs danced with the King in the dress that shone like the stars. He was determined not to lose her this time and slipped a gold ring on to her finger while they were dancing, cleverly so that she didn't notice. He tried to hold on to her at the end of the dance, but she slipped away, back to her little den and the task of making his soup. This time she put her golden reel in the bowl.

When the King found the golden reel, he sent for her again. Not having time to change, she flung the cloak of furs over her dress. As she came into the royal presence, the King caught sight of a white hand wearing the ring he had put on it as they were dancing. He grasped her hand and, when she struggled to escape, the coat opened a little, revealing the shining dress of stars. Then he tore off her cloak and hood, revealing her golden hair in all its beauty. After that she gave up trying to hide and washed the soot from her face. The King and all the court could see that she was the most beautiful woman on Earth.

Then the King said, 'You are my true bride and we will never be parted.' A marriage was arranged and they lived happily for the rest of their lives.

THE THREE FEATHERS

German Fairytale, Grimm

There was once a King who had three sons. The two elder sons were considered to be wise and handsome, but the third and youngest said very little and they called him Simple.

As the King grew older, he could not choose who would rule the kingdom after him. He decided to send each of the princes on an expedition to find a carpet. Whoever returned with the finest would rule after the King's death. He told them that each would cast a feather into the air, and whichever way the feather blew, in that direction the son would follow.

The first son offered his feather to the wind and it was taken eastwards, so he set out. The second son found his feather borne off in a westerly direction and followed it. Simple was bitterly disappointed, because no wind took his feather up and it fell lightly downwards. His direction was to remain where the feather had fallen.

Simple sat on the ground by his feather. 'How can I find a carpet from this grass that surrounds me?' he thought. As he ran his fingers through the stalks, his hand hit on something hard, and just before him was a trap door. He moved towards it and lifted it up. A flight of steps led down into the earth and took him to a little door, behind which he could hear voices. He knocked, and an old woman frog welcomed him and asked him what he needed. He told her about the carpet, and she called out to the little frogs around her, sending for her bag and drawing from it a carpet which was exquisite in colour and in texture. Simple thanked the frog and made his way back to the King. His brothers had made no effort. One had purchased an old piece of rug and the other had brought a sack cloth, but when they saw Simple's carpet it was clear he must be King.

The brothers requested a further competition. So the King told them to cast their feathers and this time bring back the most beautiful ring in the land. And they did as before, one to the west, one to the east, and one fluttering downwards, to the underneath. Simple descended the steps again and knocked at the door, and told the old frog about his need for a ring so special that none could rival its glory. She sent for her large bag and drew out a ring which sparkled with stones and diamonds. This she gave happily to Simple who thanked her and returned to his father. The elder sons were still chuckling at Simple's second fate with the feather. They forgot his former success and had put themselves to no trouble. They merely removed plated rings from a horse's harness and had returned with these. As soon as the King saw Simple's ring, he said, 'The kingdom belongs to my youngest son.'

But still the elder brothers would not submit and they begged their father to set a last competition. It was agreed that whoever could bring home the most beautiful woman would be given the kingdom. The feathers led one brother to the west, the second to the east, and Simple's feather fell effortlessly to ground on which he stood.

A third time, Simple descended the stairs to the frog and made known his request. The frog looked thoughtful and said, 'I have no such woman, but you will have one.' She gave him a carrot which had been scooped out and harnessed to six little mice. Simple accepted the gift but said, 'What am I to make of this?' The frog told him to catch one of her little frogs and sit her inside the carrot. This he did, with more than a little difficulty, but as soon it was done the frog turned into a lovely young woman, and the carrot became a golden coach, while the six little mice turned into six prancing horses. Simple kissed the maiden and returned with her to his father.

The two other brothers, quite forgetting the beautiful carpet and the glorious ring, still could not believe that Simple would succeed. Taking no more trouble than before, they chose two handsome peasant women. When the King saw Simple's woman in the coach he said, 'Without any doubt my kingdom goes to Simple, my youngest son.'

But the elder brothers, using all their cunning, deafened his ears, saying, 'Simple cannot be King. Give us one more trial. Set up a hoop in the hall for each of the women to leap through.' Wearily, the old King consented.

The peasant maidens jumped first, but one was so heavy that she broke her arm, while the other was so uncoordinated that she snapped a leg. The Frog Princess sprung as lightly as a deer through the hoop! There could be no deterring the King. The youngest brother married the woman who loved him dearly, and, after his father's death, they ruled the land with wisdom and equity, for many years.

THE THREE LITTLE PIGS
English Fairytale

An old woman had three little pigs that ate and ate and became so fat that they could hardly fit into their sty. One day she said to them, 'You can't stay here with me any longer. Go away and build your own houses!'

So the three little pigs went out to begin their life in the big, wide world.

The first little pig met a man with a bundle of straw and said to him, 'Please, sir, will you give me some of your straw so that I can build myself a house?'

The man replied, 'Gladly, if you will give me some of your bristles to make a brush.'

The little pig gave him some bristles and the man gave him some straw and helped him to build a house with a big door at the front and a little door at the back. Then the little pig moved in, saying to himself, 'If the big wolf comes, I'll be safe inside.'

The second little pig met a man carrying a bundle of wood and said to him, 'Please, sir, give me some wood so that I can build a house.' And the man said, 'Gladly, if you will give me some bristles to make myself a brush.' The exchange was made and the man helped him to build a wooden house with a big door at the front and a little door at the back. And the pig felt safe inside.

The third little pig met a man pushing a cart full of stones. He asked for some stones and the man asked for some bristles and helped him to build a house of stone with a big door at the front and a little door at the back. And the pig felt safe inside.

Now all the little pigs were living in houses of their own. The wolf heard about this and he came out of the forest. He came to the house of straw and knocked at the big front door, calling out, 'Little pig, little pig, let me in!'

The little pig called back, 'No, no, by the hair of my chinny chin chin, I'll not let you in.'

The wolf said, 'Then I'll huff and I'll puff and I'll blow your house down!' He huffed and he puffed and the straw house came tumbling down. But the little pig was nowhere to be seen because he had run out of the little door at the back and gone to take refuge with the second little pig, whose house was made of wood.

Then the wolf went to the wooden house, knocked on the front door and called out, 'Little pig, little pig, let me in!' The second little pig called back 'No, no, by the hair of my chinny chin chin, I'll not let you in.' 'Then,' said the wolf, 'I'll blow your house down!'

And he huffed and he puffed and he blew the house down. But by then the two little pigs had escaped through the little door at the back and taken refuge with the third little pig, whose house was made of stone.

The wolf came to the stone house and called out, 'Little pig, little pig, let me in.' The little pig called back, 'No, no, by the hair of my chinny chin chin, I'll not let you in.' And the wolf said, 'Then I'll huff and I'll puff and I'll blow the house down!'

He huffed and he puffed, but nothing happened. Going round the back of the house, he started to climb on the roof. His plan was to climb down the chimney and catch them all. But the three little pigs lit a big fire and heated up a cauldron of boiling water. When the wolf came sliding down the chimney into the pot, they clapped on the lid and danced around it, singing, 'Hurrah, hurrah, the big bad wolf is dead!' Then the first two little pigs built themselves houses of stone and they all lived happily ever after.

TIDDALIK THE FROG
Native Australian

Tiddalik was a very big frog. He lived in the Dreamtime and he was huge, like a mountain. One day he was very thirsty. He opened his mouth and drank up all the rain as it fell from the sky, but still he was thirsty. So he looked around and began to drink the water from all the pools and the streams and the rivers.

The other creatures of the Dreamtime saw that the land was drying up. The plants and trees were dying of thirst. The animals were getting thirstier and thirstier. They all became very frightened. The drought was killing everything except Tiddalik, the enormous frog, who was growing bigger and bigger. Then the animals realised where the water had gone. It was all inside Tiddalik.

The animals called a meeting. They spoke of only one thing. How could they get Tiddalik to open his mouth and give the water back to the land? He was so big and so powerful. Some of the animals despaired, saying there was nothing to be done and they were all going to die. Then the Wombat had an idea. He said, 'What we have to do is make Tiddalik laugh. If he laughs, he will have to open his mouth!'

The other animals agreed. They would go and visit Tiddalik and see if they could make him laugh. They went to the place where he sat, resting with his eyes closed and his huge belly full of water. They all gathered round him and each animal in turn did its best to make him laugh.

Kookaburra went first. He laughed his famous, infectious laugh, but Tiddalik didn't even smile. He took no notice at all.

Then Kangaroo hopped and jumped around Tiddalik, performing a cabaret. This made all the other animals laugh, but not Tiddalik. He just sat there.

Then Lizard tried, making his quick, darting movements. Tiddalik just sat there, solemn and unblinking, his mouth tight shut.

At last Naburnum, the eel, came slithering across the parched earth and placed himself carefully in front of Tiddalik. He caught the frog's eye with a steady gaze and raised himself off the ground until he was balancing on his tail. Then he began to sway from side to side. It was the beginning of his dance and Tiddalik was watching.

At first Naburnum danced gently and calmly. The frog was mesmerised. Gradually, the eel's movements got wilder, twisting and turning into the funniest shapes. Tiddalik's eyes gleamed with pleasure. He held his belly and for a while he managed not to laugh. But he couldn't take his eyes off Naburnum jumping and wriggling and squirming. At last his mouth began to twitch and suddenly it opened. Tiddalik laughed. As he laughed, all the waters of the world gushed out. The big streams filled up with beautiful, clear water. Every pond and stream was filled. The plants began to grow again and the animals were no longer thirsty.

That was how Naburnum the eel saved the world, but it was the Wombat's idea. And it happened in the Dreamtime.

THE TWIN WARRIOR HEROES

Native American

There were once twin warriors who had walked a holy trail, but the time had come for them to move on and make their way to the house of their great father, the Sun. So they set out.

Seeing smoke arising, they made their way down into the Cavern of old Spider Woman who asked them where they were going. She warned them of dangers on the road and gave them two gifts. One was a life feather, and the second, a prayer to go with them to prevent danger. She made them learn it:

Put pollen on your head,
Put pollen on your hands,
Put pollen on your feet,
Be still.

She was right, for danger is always close. The warriors fell into rocks that crushed their bodies, then reeds that cut their limbs, and cacti that tore their skin, while underneath there was sand which burned their feet. Each time, they said their prayer and the danger stilled and they past safely through.

The gates to the House of the Sun were guarded by two fierce bears. The boys stilled them with their prayer and passed through. They knocked at the door and were let into the house by Sky Woman. She told them to fear their father, who would soon be home, and she wrapped them up in a sky cloth for safety and placed them on a shelf.

When he arrived, the Sun sensed the warriors hidden in their cloth and pulled them down from the shelf. He half-believed their claim to be his sons, but wanted to test them to see. First, he cast them on to a spike, but they used the life feather and were saved. He threw them overnight into a fiery sweat lodge, but the life feather looked after them, and he found them well in the morning. Finally, he chose to smoke a pipe with them, filling it with poisoned tobacco. But a caterpillar came invisibly to them, offering a tiny stone and advising them to suck on it as they smoked. So they took of the pipe, and were none the worse – in fact, it seemed as if they even enjoyed it.

At this, the Great Sun acknowledged they were his sons. He offered them a place beside him and made all his resources available. But they could not stay, for their work had only begun, and if the trail ahead had danger, it certainly also offered a balance of richness and beauty.

WATER JAR BOY, CHILDHOOD
——OF THE HUMAN HERO——
Pueblo Indian

A young Pueblo woman, who was helping her mother mix clay for pottery with her foot, felt a splash of mud on her leg, but thought no more of it. After some days the girl felt something was moving in her belly, but she did not think anything about having a baby. She did not tell her mother. But it was growing and growing.

One day in the morning she was very sick. In the afternoon she got the baby. Then her mother knew, for the first time, about her daughter's baby. The mother was very angry about it, but after she looked at the baby she saw it was not like a baby. She saw it was a round thing with two things sticking out – it was a little jar. 'Where did you get this?' said her mother. The girl was just crying. About that time the father came in. 'Never mind, I am very glad she had a baby,' he said. 'But it's not a baby!' said her mother. Then the father went to look at it and saw it was a little water jar. After that he was very fond of that water jar. 'It's moving,' he said. Pretty soon that little jar was growing. In twenty days it was big. It was able to go round with the children, and it could talk. 'Grandfather, take me outdoors so I can look around,' he said.

So every morning the grandfather would take him out and the children would play with him and they became fond of him. They found out he was a boy, Water Jar Boy. They found out from his talking.

One day the men were going out to hunt rabbits, and Water Jar Boy wanted to go. 'Grandfather, could you take me down to the foot of the mesa? I want to hunt rabbits.'

'Poor grandson, you can't hunt rabbits, you have no legs or arms,' said the grandfather. But Water Jar Boy was very anxious to go. 'Take me anyway. You are too old, and you can't do anything.' His mother was crying because her boy had no arms or legs or eyes.

So next morning his grandfather took him down to the south on the flat. Then he rolled along, and pretty soon a rabbit ran out and he began to chase it. Just before he got to the marsh there was a rock. He hit himself against it and broke, and a boy jumped up. He was very glad his skin had been broken and that he was a boy, a big boy. He was wearing lots of beads around his neck and turquoise earrings, and a dance kilt and moccasins, and a buckskin shirt. Catching a number of rabbits, he returned and presented them to his grandfather, who brought him triumphantly home.

WHISKY JACK
Native Canadian

Hundreds of years ago there lived a powerful chieftain and medicine man whose name was Whisky Jack. He had three wolves for blood brothers and they were his constant companions, keeping him warm with their fur in winter and fanning him with their tails in the heat of the summer. He was widely respected and his magic powers protected his tribe against many dangers. When the land was covered by a great flood, he saved his people and all living creatures by taking them on to a huge stone raft that he made when he saw the danger coming.

Whisky Jack was very proud of his great powers. As time went on, he became arrogant and boastful. One day he was standing on the shore of Lake Superior, throwing rocks into the water and boasting, 'I am the greatest. I am all-powerful!'

At that moment a rock he had just thrown hit Mishipeshu, the water god, on the nose. Now, if you knew Mishipeshu, you would know that was not a good thing to do. Mishipeshu was furious. Moments later the waters parted and a huge trout sprang towards Whisky Jack, swallowing him in one great gulp.

Whisky Jack found himself sloshing around in the stomach of the huge fish. It was dark and wet and slippery in there. For once, the chieftain felt weak and powerless. He was unsteady on his feet and became very seasick as the great fish lurched from side to side in the water.

But he didn't give up hope. His eyes got used to the darkness and he had an idea. He had left his bow and arrows behind on the shore, but his knife was still tucked into his belt. With it, he sliced a small hole through the monster's stomach. He saw the ribs arching above him. Chipping and slicing, he managed to cut loose one of those great, arching bones and sharpened it at the end. Then he listened for the beating of the heart and with all his strength he thrust the spear towards it.

The great fish thrashed violently in the water and eventually floated, dead, to the surface of the lake. Whisky Jack climbed up into its throat, thinking to escape through its mouth. He found the jaws tightly locked. There was no way out and Whisky Jack knew that he was defeated, that he would die unless someone rescued him. He knelt down and prayed to the great god Manitou, asking for help.

Manitou heard his prayer and sent a flock of ravens that alighted on the body of the great fish and began to peck away its flesh. After a while, Whisky Jack saw specks of light appearing and growing bigger until he could see the water of the lake and the shore beyond. He was inside a floating skeleton. With his knife, Whisky Jack carved out one of the great teeth and made it into a paddle. Then he paddled his strange skeleton boat towards the shore.

The people saw the skeleton of the great fish travelling towards them paddled by Whisky Jack and they gathered round, praising him as the greatest. But Whisky Jack knew better and, to show them, he turned himself into an ordinary jack rabbit. After that, whenever he felt the temptation to be high and mighty, he would turn himself into a rabbit, reminding himself that, in the eyes of the great god Manitou, all creatures are equal and a chieftain is no better than a jack rabbit.

THE WHITE SNAKE

German Fairytale, Grimm

A special dish is brought by a servant for an old King each night. One night, the servant looks into the dish and sees a white snake. He tastes it and hears strange whispering. The snake has given him the power of understanding the language of animals and birds.

One day, the Queen loses her gold ring, and suspicion falls on the servant. The King threatens with angry words – unless the servant finds the thief, he will be executed on the morrow.

The servant goes into the courtyard, where he hears ducks. He hears one duck say that he has swallowed the Queen's ring. The servant seizes the duck and takes him to the kitchen.

The Queen's ring is recovered.

The King grants him a favour. The servant asks for a horse and money to go travelling.

On his travels, the servant comes to water. He sees three fish caught in the reeds, gasping. He puts them back in the water. The fish are delighted. They will remember and repay.

He rides on. He hears ants talking in the sand at his feet. They complain that heavy hoofs have been treading down their people. The servant turns on his path. The ants say they will remember and repay.

He goes into a wood. Two old ravens are standing at their nest and throwing out their young. They cry, 'We shall starve.' The servant kills his horse and gives it to them. They will remember: one good turn deserves another.

He arrives at a city and sees a crowd. A messenger is saying that the King's daughter wants a husband. Suitors must complete a task or be executed.

The servant becomes a suitor. A gold ring is thrown into the sea, and he is ordered to fetch the ring. Alone in the sea, three fishes bring him the ring. He takes it to the King.

The Princess is not satisfied he is her equal, and another task is set. Ten sacks of millet seed are strewn on the grass. They are to be picked up by daybreak. The ants come to his aid.

The Princess still cannot conquer her proud heart. She wants an apple from the tree of life. The two ravens in the wood knock down the apple. The servant and the Princess cut the apple and eat it together. They are happy.

Appendix

Story Notes

These notes offer some information about the stories that may be of interest and of use, as well as a few specific exercises that have evolved in working with individual stories as myth enactments. The notes vary in length and content, the length or brevity of a note being in no way an indicator of the story's importance. Their purpose is never to be prescriptive, bearing in mind that the essence of the Sesame approach is for the individual therapist to construct sessions out of his or her own relation to the story, with material that feels comfortable and authentic. Rather, they can be thought of as jumping-off points from which to devise myth sessions that will work, imaginatively, for you and for the group you are working with.

We have included some outstanding exercises that feel important to us, personally, from myth sessions in our experience, either as participants or when leading a session. These may be described quite graphically. Other exercises may not sound so good, but will come into their own 'in the doing'. As ever, when devising drama, the way to decide if you want to use an exercise is to try it out and see how it feels.

Information about the stories themselves is offered serendipitously, as we have felt moved to include it, again in the expectation that every therapist who works with the stories will research their background and discover other details that may feel equally important or relevant to them.

Abu Kasem's Slippers

Humour is sometimes the medicine people need. The story of *Abu Kasem's Slippers* has an inbuilt humour that doesn't require work. The more seriously it is played, the funnier it gets. Yet, underneath the humour, it is quite a serious story.

Akinidi and the Coming of Happiness

This story came to us through Margaret Leona, a storyteller and vice-president of Sesame, who found it in James Riordan's *The Sun Maiden and the Cresent Moon: Siberian Folk Tales*. It is the quintessential story of the arts therapies in action, with people finding happiness through participation in singing, dancing and pattern making. At the same time, it allows a place for the darker side of human nature to be expressed. People welcome the chance to invoke a witch in the midst of a happy scene and be destructive within the boundaries of drama.

Akinidi is a useful enactment story at all sorts of times. It can be a good way to end a series of story sessions because of the imperative it carries about the power and expression of joy over loss, and what seems like the ending of death. A ceremony can be held after the story is enacted where an Akinidi candle is lit, representing the light and commitment to the creative, to song and to dance. Each person is given the chance to light their own night light while making a movement or speaking a sentence to ask for what they need from that light for their own well-being and creativity. The group can then talk about how this might be implemented.

Ali Baba and the Forty Thieves

This is the story from *The Arabian Nights* from which Sesame takes its name. It is often used as a means of introducing the Sesame approach to people, because the central motif of unlocking a treasure cave is quickly recognisable, offering a metaphor for the relationship between inner and outer consciousness.

After the story has been told, the enactments can be worked in small groups of four or five people. Each group may be asked to come up with three sculpts of the story, or, if ready, a full enactment, which is run through and then shared with the other groups. The final part of the enactment can be done through everyone spontaneously embodying the treasure in the cave, first non-verbally and then adding words.

It is a very useful story for enabling people to think obliquely about restriction and potential.

Amaterasu the Sun Goddess

In recent years this Japanese story has become popular with Sesame students in training. Clearly, something attracts them towards the idea of a goddess being driven into hiding and having to be coaxed out into the world again. The mirror theme offers ideas for *bridges in* and *out*. Or the strong open and closed motif can be worked in movement or exercises of the imagination.

Ash

The character of Ash is a good example of the counter-hero. He is passive, Zen-like or contemplative, waiting for something to happen, unlike the more assertive heroes who gird up their egos and take on challenges through obstacle-laden journeys.

The story is particularly useful for seated groups where energy in the client group is low. This tale honours slowness. The enactment can be worked round the edges of the group, with help from the Sesame practitioner in the centre when Ash moves into his more enlivened moments of overcoming conflict.

When this story was worked with hyperactive children, they were always contained by the final image of Ash, lying on his back and bearing the weight of the world on a pole, which he manages to balance. He is the only being with the stillness, strength and magic to bear the weight of the sky and keep the world in place.

A *bridge in* can work in twos, playing with different qualities and energy in movement, developing these and then exploring their opposites. Exercises using phrases like 'Hurry up' and 'Slow down' can also be worked with.

The Bad People

Stories have a way of appearing when they are needed. This one emerged in the course of ongoing work with a group of children who had suffered physical and emotional abuse. Marian Lindkvist was working with the Sesame team at that time and came in one day with the story scribbled in pencil on a piece of paper. Enacting it was almost like playing a game, yet the symbolism of the stolen treasure strikes deep. The children asked for it again and again. Though it is not a traditional story, it became part of the tradition in that particular place. We have included it because it worked so well.

Beauty and the Beast

Both adults and children find this familiar story exciting to enact because of the relationship that develops between the polarity of the vulnerable, unblemished feminine and the unacceptable masculine, cursed with a hidden enchantment. The stolen rose and the healing tear are powerful motifs that give the story potency.

Working with a well-established group, the *bridge in* could play with the idea of hidden distortions or shapes. This can be done by asking the group to walk round the room holding, for example, a heel, or walking on the outside of a foot, so that the appearance and movement are out of the ordinary. In this way Beast qualities begin to be explored.

If the group is secure, this exercise can be developed so that people work in pairs. A can sit down with a percussion instrument in hand. B joins A back to back. The aim of the exercise is for A to 'woo' B into becoming visible. B can remain hidden if he/she wishes. The exercise is reversed and then discussed before going into the story.

The Boy who Lived with Bears

The boy's song when he is walled up in the cave is an important turning point in this story. It therefore needs to be prepared for in advance with some confidence-building voice warm-ups and a suitable phrase or two of song that the boy can use, supported by one or two people in the background. A little group of children in a care home loved the part of the story where the boy makes his home with bears, rolling about in their cave in mock fights with his bear brothers.

Cap-o'-Rushes

Using this story, the Sesame team worked with Simon, a boy aged nine living in a therapeutic community. Simon had been sexually abused by his mother and often behaved violently at the end of dramatherapy sessions, attacking the female therapists. He had great strength.

So that Simon could take part in *Cap-o'-Rushes*, we transposed the sexes, a Queen instead of a King and a son instead of a daughter. During the enactment, when it came to the part where the Queen realises that she is remembering the son she sent away, the therapist playing the Queen role began to cry, saying, 'Now I understand. How cruel and stupid I have been. I sent him away for saying that he loved me as salt loves meat, but now I know that he really loved me. Oh, how I wish I could find him and tell him how sorry I am.'

Then Cap-o'-Rushes (Simon) stood before her and said, 'I am here, Mother!' And the Queen recognised him and hugged him and said, 'It's you. It is really you. I am so sorry for what I did.'

Simon played the part of the youngest son with complete concentration and feeling. When the Queen wept at the wedding feast because she had lost her son, Simon stepped forward in role and comforted her. He was at once in role and totally himself. He said, 'It's all right, Mum. I love you, Mum. I love you.' He flung himself into her arms and hugged her and repeated over and over, 'I love you, Mum. I really love you.'

The moment was real, but it was held by the story form. We were all close to tears. The three of us then had the task of containing these powerful feelings within the drama.

Cap-o'-Rushes/Simon was able to introduce his Mother Queen to the Princess he was about to marry. He did this without prompting, saying, 'This is my wife.'

The story ended with us all in role and a good grounding followed, so that people were back to themselves for the end of the session. Simon was able to leave the room this time without attacking anyone or his usual reluctance to return to his own world. He simply called, 'See you next week,' and made his way back to his room.

Chiron the Wounded Healer

This ancient descent story is developed from Michael Kearney's telling in his book *Mortally Wounded*.[1] The story has been used many times when working with therapists, because it speaks directly to the reality, often denied, that the one who offers healing frequently joins a healing profession as a means of resolving her or his own unresolved pain.

To many, naming this is a relief. The story turns the idea of the therapist being the expert upside down and offers a place for 'wounding' to be worked mutually, client and therapist together.

The end of the myth is sometimes questioned after enactment. Is Zeus' rescue from Tartarus, the deepest, darkest part of the underworld, a cop-out? Is being raised to the heavens in a constellation of stars a desirable change? Who is to say?

---

1   Kearney 1986.

In astrology charts, the comet Chiron represents how the deepest wound affects other parts of a person's life. Chiron gives meaning to pain. Esoteric studies would argue that Chiron's presence in the heavens continues to guide those who look to the stars and planets for wisdom.

It is interesting that Tartarus, a prison in Hades, becomes for many enactors a place where they find peace and newness. Many who have been anxious to visit the underworld in role report that, after an imaginary visit, they want to stay there. They find that the unknown has befriended them and they return more confident to trust.

The story works well as a sound enactment, with the roles being sounded or sung. A thorough voice warm-up is required for this form of enactment and the Sesame practitioner needs to be confident in holding a space for voice work.

The story is not suitable if the group members are insecure with one another or not yet ready to consider the potential of shadow.

A client writes about working with Chiron:

> As the story was being told, I felt like Chiron. I was like him. His leg and the pain I feel seemed to become one. I had no hope. I realised I needed the underworld because, somewhere, I know that underneath place.

> The release of Prometheus made me think of men in my life who were consumed and punished by things. Their attitude had affected me. I realised as I made my way down to Tartarus that this was the first visit to meeting deep, unmet parts of myself which I have covered up until now.

> Like Chiron, I knew it was OK to take time and let the 'shades' say what would happen next. I gave up planning for a bit and trusted something else to take over.

Coyote and the Land of the Dead

People who struggle with unresolved grieving are often drawn to this story. It really engages with that territory, while allowing space for participants in the enactment to enter the experience on their own terms. A young woman who had been unable to reconcile herself to her father's death took the part of Eagle and played it with great concentration, taking the enactment very slowly. Her facial expression in role was bleak and still. She really became Eagle. Enactment in such circumstances goes way beyond acting. The experience of catharsis in the final separation from Eagle Woman and others who did not want to return to the land of the living was felt by the whole group.

Alida Gersie writes about this story at some length in her sensitive book *Storymaking in Bereavement: Dragons Fight in the Meadow.*[2]

Creation Myth of the Mayans

Creation stories like this one, *Eurynome and the Egg of the Cosmos, In the Beginning* and *Kaang* address questions about how the world was made, how humanity came into being and the relationship between the creators and the created. All peoples have a story of their land and race, symbolic narratives which must be understood in terms of the culture. This particular story looks closely at the creating divinity having a stormy relationship with humankind.

Demeter and Persephone

This is another huge story, a myth of descent, loss and initiation, to name just three of its themes, which requires a long session or two to get the best out of it. However, in a clinical setting it can be used without the details, keeping the focus on Persephone's story.

Elidore

At some level, Elidore could be seen as the dyslexic hero. He cannot remember his lessons and fails at school. So he takes himself away and finds himself through a different education. There he succeeds because the standard of the new land is achievable for him. The pedagogy of imagination is something that children and adults are seldom offered as a complement or opposite to linear learning. Elidore is given this chance and it opens up his capacity for intuitive thinking. Children love this story and enjoy using *gobbledygook* as the language of the country on the other side of the cave.

Eurynome and the Egg of the Cosmos

This is a useful starting story.

The egg-cracking motif and the things that tumble out can be very powerful for people. The simplicity of the story belies the universal

---

2   Gersie 1991.

symbol of new life. Watch out for the enactment end! Make sure that sufficient time for the *bridge out* is given.

An example of the *bridge out* is for people to imagine their own egg, seeing its shape and colour. They can be asked to check out if the egg needs to stay whole, or if there is a crack ready to open to hatch something. This can be shown in a movement, with a short time given for anyone who wants to speak to what they see in words. People normally find something new is waiting for them.

The Flowering Tree

This beautiful story comes from Pat. We do not know where she found it, but with its motifs of the child seeing what the adults miss or deny, there is a familiarity with Jumping Mouse – the call of the river and a breaking away from the collective to attend to what is uniquely waiting to be found. It is in an individuation story of supply.

Forever-Mountain

An angry eight-year-old boy made this story his own and returned to it every session for the best part of a year. It was the first story he would consent to work with, having spent many sessions beating up and 'killing' imaginary opponents in a soft play room. These solitary fights were gradually turned into formal boxing and karate matches with the therapist as referee, but all stories were rejected.

When the story of Forever-Mountain was offered, that was another matter. The Sumi wrestler was the perfect role model, already strong and with three very strong women giving their full attention to making him invincible. With the therapist in role as the grandmother, he was prepared to stop beating up the soft play and learn the cut and thrust of 'shadow boxing', with a no-touching rule to keep things safe. Dramatic enactment of the story gave a shape to his aggression and focused him in a more positive way. The story was repeated and repeated. At the end of the last session of the year, with Forever-Mountain and his young wife living in their new house, he put words to what the story had given him: 'I'm the strongest man of all, aren't I? And if anyone tries to hurt my wife, I can defend her, can't I?'

The Great White Bird

This story from the Bushmen of the Kalahari works beautifully as a dance movement piece, essentially for two people, though there is room for others in very minor roles, being questioned as the hunter travels in search of the bird. To avoid self-consciousness, the dance enactment can be set up with the group divided into pairs, working at the same time in different parts of the room. Accompanying sound can be with instruments and voice, or a suitable piece of recorded music.

The Handless Maiden

This story has great appeal to contemporary fiction writers and poets, including Margaret Atwood and Anne Sexton, who have produced their own versions of it, and the theme has been taken up in cinema and theatre, a recent version being Kneehigh Theatre's production *The Wild Bride*. The motif of the girl's hands being severed by her father is often felt as a reference to the physical abuse of women. The story also has resonances of sexual abuse by the father, as in the Grimm's story of *Thousandfurs*. Offering it for enactment does not, of course, require the dramatherapist to know what it is about. That is the beauty of these myths and fairytales. They offer an experience which every participant is free to feel and interpret in his or her own way, according to how it feels in the doing. That way the story never loses its capacity to surprise.

The Healing Herb

This is a story out of Sesame's oral tradition. It fits with a common experience when working with emotionally damaged children who, on entering into a story in a group situation, will sometimes produce spontaneous sub-stories in which they are symbolically asking for attention and help. Going on a journey, for example, the child will 'fall' and be found to have broken a leg. This requires a slight diversion within the story to bring the child back into the action. The story of *The Healing Herb* stays with this need for healing as a theme for a whole session and has been used as such in clinical settings where this need comes to the fore.

The Holy Grail

The Holy Grail is a long and mystical Celtic story. It needs to be done as a series rather than rushed in a one-hour session. It has as its central theme a quest for the Grail chalice, found out of an all-encompassing wasteland. It considers a place for the thirst of the soul wound to be tended. The Holy Grail cup is an early version of the cup of Christ. It is free from the trammels of en-churched religion but speaks to the soul by asking two questions: 'What ails thee?' and 'Whom does the Grail serve?'

A participant writes:

> I recall the pivotal part of the Holy Grail day was when we were taken to the 'Wasteland' during the *bridge in*. I remember ending up on my knees connecting with my weariness, but it was when it was suggested that we give voice that I wholly connected to 'my pain'. This was the key indicator to being ready to explore greater depths.

> I found some kind of edge or boundary and with ready curiosity I momentarily crossed over and allowed myself to feel my suffering self. In that moment, I felt pain and comfort. A letting out. I was always 'feeling for others' but felt shame when it came to myself. I could not write about it – but I did draw a picture. Now when I write I see it was the beginning of me exploring how to be my own good mother. I have always cared for the world and from that experience, in very simple terms, I began to take a compassionate interest in me.

A member of the clergy and *Holy Grail* enactor writes:

> I don't think we can understand the longing which comes around the Grail cup, but it is good to know it is part of our soul story – that somewhere beneath the pain of the longing there is an active energy. You can never get to this through thinking.

> Because of the pain, ego has to shove over a bit and make space – and once you can survive that, you begin to trust that space. It's like a surrender – you give into the longing, kind of trust it. You just have to wait on inner action.

> It reminds me of that bit where the person says, 'If the person begins to respond to the psyche, then psyche responds one thousand fold.'

The Hymn of the Pearl

This is a Gnostic myth about the exile and redemption of the soul. The original text in Old Syriac is in the British Museum and the story was first published in *The Acts of Judas Thomas the Apostle* in 938 AD. The Jungian analyst Edward Edinger, referring to the story in *Ego and Archetype*, writes of it as 'a beautiful symbolic expression of the theory of analytical psychology concerning the origin and development of the conscious ego',[3] which has to go through a necessary process of separation from its original, child state and become alienated and lost, before it can achieve symbolic awareness.

In the Beginning

Another creation story. Although a myth is seldom the way to introduce enactment in a new group, a creation myth with its universal rather than personal content can be a good way to start.

Inanna in the Underworld

Along with *Chiron the Wounded Healer* and *The Mysteries of Orpheus*, this is one of the trusted descent stories in the Sesame collection. It tells of the descent of a woman to the underworld, going to meet her dark sister. The dressing of Inanna, Queen of Earth and Heaven, and the subsequent removal of her riches until she stands naked in the underworld is a stark and strong image, which can be felt to represent disempowerment, bereavement, grief, exile, humiliation for many.

A client writes about *Inanna*:

> The story is beautiful and it is cruel. It holds the hardness of the price that has to be paid in order to go from 'the great above to the great below' – and then come back.

> Going down into the unconscious is a process and maybe that is why it has seven gates – seven choices to be made. You have to check if you are ready at each stage – you are paying a price. The gatekeeper is very demanding but has to demand the cost.

Inanna in the Underworld is the most frequently told and performed part of the much longer Sumerian myth of *Inanna*, believed to be the oldest written story in the world, going back over 4000 years and probably predating *The Epic of Gilgamesh*. It was inscribed on fragmented cuneiform tablets, recovered by archaeologists from sites at Nipur and Ur of the Chaldees. The whole story of *Inanna* was put together and retranslated by Samuel Kramer, the expert on ancient Sumer, and published in a full and beautiful version, in collaboration with the storyteller Diane Wolkstein.[4]

---

3   Edinger 1972, p.121.
4   Wolkstein and Kramer 1983.

Inanna in the Underworld has a long history in the oral tradition of Sesame and was being used for Sesame enactments before publication of this book, though some echoes of Wolkstein's language have crept in. It is a powerful story, requiring at least half a day for a group to become thoroughly immersed and to emerge safely from its impact.[5]

It helps to *bridge in* to the full enactment with some ritual exercises, which may include:

1. Working in pairs, one person takes the part of Inanna and the other, her servant Ninshibur, for a slow and formal robing of the Queen in the seven *mē*, the garments of her power.

2. Divide into two or more groups. In different parts of the room, each group embodies seven different gates. The gates are shown by each of the groups in turn.

Iron Hans

This story of the wild man at the bottom of the lake and a boy working his way towards manhood is the theme of the book *Iron John*, in which Robert Bly explores the symbolism of the story in his quest for 'new visions of what a man is or could be'.[6] Bly's starting point, when he was running his famous men's groups and writing the book in the 1980s, was that men were becoming aware that 'the images of adult manhood given by the popular culture are worn out'.[7] Like Marion Woodman, Bly is of great interest to Sesame practitioners because he works with his groups in a practical, physical way, drawing on Jung's psychology and the inherited wisdom of fairytales. This is another big story, needing at least half a day and, ideally, a whole weekend to enact.

Jumping Mouse

At first read, *Jumping Mouse* appears to be a children's story because the characters are creatures rather than people. However, the story theme is the hero's journey told in symbols which, although set in a Native American landscape, are cross-cultural and can be universally understood by young and old enactors.

Jumping Mouse addresses the subject of leaving home to attend to what Joseph Campbell means when he advocates that a person *follows their*

---

5   See Perera 1981.
6   Bly 1990, p.ix.
7   Bly 1990, p.303.

bliss. It can be seen as a story of individuation. The transformation which comes at the end, when Mouse becomes Eagle, is always shocking. In telling this story before enactment, there is always a bemused moment at the end, when the significance of mouse becoming his predator sinks in. It is a moment that challenges ego thinking.

Within Native American culture, the Eagle represents strength, courage and wisdom. Eagle can rise above the material to see the spiritual. Eagle signifies power, balance, intuition and a grace of creative spirit, achieved through knowledge and hard work. The experience of this comes when the story is enacted.

A fun way into the story is to play with imaginary names. What would your name be if you could change it today? How would that name move you and enable you to meet others?

A *bridge out* works well when you ask people to imagine Jumping Mouse as Eagle. What would being Eagle be like for him? What would he do with his Eagle power? What would that power make of him?

Kaang

This story of Kaang with the great tree between the upper and lower worlds has been written about earlier in the book. It holds important themes about rules and regulations and when to break them.

A client writes:

> Before the story we had to choose a card with a tree and I found mine easily. I chose one with a huge middle, trunk and roots. As I did this, I found a relationship between the roots of the tree and my own stomach. This let me understand the connection between the roots of a person and the memory of trauma. I realised the crucial role of the stomach as a central container to what had gone before. In this moment I found a connection between roots of the tree image and the nervous system in the stomach.

> When the therapist said that the tree would give me a gift after the story, I found that it gave me breath. That's the only thing I needed at that time. I breathed and freed my stomach and leg-roots.

King Laurin

A festive story with a difference and a touch of magic, making a change at Christmas time. Can be rounded off with real clementines and mince pies as a grounding if Christmas is very near.

Korozuka

Pat worked with this story when teaching Myths on the Sesame course and it is one that needs to be used carefully. As in *Prince Ring*, there is an unopened cupboard, but in this one there is no helpful symbol of the shadow. In this story, the content of the cupboard, like a Bluebeard's locked room, is demonic. The story can be told up to the part where the servant looks inside, and then in the enactment the group members are left to come up with ideas of what he saw.

This story has been used in a long-standing and ongoing Sesame group where there was a lot of trust between group members. A great deal of time was spent in the *bridge out* discussing the relationship between the sweet old woman and the flesh and bones.

The Lion, the Young Man and the Black Storm Tree

This Bushmen myth has a mysterious power which plays with the emotions in a way that can be upsetting. The lion licking the young hunter's tears suggests a tenderness which in no way prefigures the ending in death of the boy and the lion.

The Little Earth Cow

The theme of a magical, nurturing animal which looks after young people who have suffered neglect and abuse recurs in European fairytales. So does the theme of the kind child who responds to the magic and is nurtured by it, while the bad child is not. The nurturing of Gretel in her secret home by the little Earth Cow has warm potential for enactment, but the second half of the story, with the butchering of the Earth Cow, is strong medicine, to be introduced and contained with care.

Loki and Baldur

This is a dark and shocking story. The confident, cocky young Baldur, who believes himself to be protected by his mother's magic, is killed by the machinations of Loki, an envious trickster. The worst part is that the fatal blow is struck by a blind brother in the belief that Baldur cannot be harmed. A group of storytellers, enacting the story at a conference, commented on how different the story felt as a result of experiencing it in an embodied way.

The Magic Drum

This Inuit story of the girl who refuses to marry and goes on a perilous, transformative journey is one of the relatively few hero's journeys in which the hero is a woman.

Mella

This Shero journey story works well as a sound enactment. It takes a lot of facilitation by the Sesame practitioner to enable a group to sing/sound a spontaneous storytelling. Mella lends itself well to this with the two main themes of arduous journey and love overcoming terror.

To set up a 'tell and sing' enactment, a lengthy body/voice warm-up with use of percussion instruments is essential before. The story-singer then invites the group to participate in the story by creating the sounds of Mella's journey using instruments and voice. The group can also be invited to come into the centre of the circle and to act out parts of the story spontaneously – for example, the healing dance of the shamans, the coiling of the serpent.

The story-singer then begins to sing the story, leaving moments for the sound-enactors to participate. The story-singer needs to lead but at the same time leave spaces so that the group members get the idea that the sound space is theirs to fill. Use of repetitive phrases which the participants recognise can be used by the story-singer – for example, 'Four long days she travelled, Four long days.' Or 'Her love for her father was greater! Oh! Her love for her father was greater.'

The Mysteries of Orpheus

The great skill of Orpheus was music. His singing and playing charmed all creation, humankind, creatures and nature alike. This gift is sorely tested when Orpheus loses his beloved who has died and has crossed over to the underworld. He fails to meet the conditions Zeus sets to bring her back which demands he must trust his music to woo her. In looking back to see her, he loses her a second time.

In his book *The Soul in Grief*,[8] Robert Romanyshyn chronicles the sudden death of his wife Janet. He likens the story of Orpheus to the grief journey that takes bereaved men and women through our own consideration of the underworld, so that a return to life is made when the mourned has been honoured. The story could well be used to work with loss issues.

The myth has various endings. Most tell of the trauma of Orpheus who is not immediately ready to let his beloved go. In some tellings, he is ripped to pieces by a band of frolicking Maenads, wild women who take him over and destroy him. In other tellings, he dies and his head is severed and thrown to a river which carries the head to Lesbos where he becomes an oracle of wisdom. In others, he wanders aimlessly singing the saddest of songs.

The Myth of Er

The Myth of Er is the story that James Hillman, founder of archetypal psychology, cites as holding the core theory for his work on Soul. It is referenced rather briefly in his book *The Soul's Code*.[9]

James Hillman became a Patron of the Sesame Institute in 2006 and came to a myth enactment of *The Myth of Er*. He did not participate but watched as a room full of people retold the story in enactment. At the end he said, 'This is amazing. This Soul thing is real.' What he saw afresh in the Sesame work was the embodiment of everything he wrote about. The quotation included earlier in this book comes from his experience on that day.

Prince Ring

This magical story was used a lot with children in a residential care setting. The hidden Snati-Snati dog in the cupboard represented a locked-away part of themselves that was always a fun way of giving the child an experience of the inner helper.

'Choose me, choose me!'

---

8   Romanyshyn 1999.
9   Hillman 1997.

The antagonist Rauder is overcome by Snati-Snati, and many times the Sesame team witnessed a child's sense of justice when the bully was exiled and the land was free for a new and fair King.

Psyche and Eros

The myth of *Psyche and Eros* is one of the best-known stories in classical Greek mythology. Psyche, a beautiful princess, personifies the human soul. She is the symbol of the soul purified by passions and trials, who gains immortality through love with Eros. It is a big story and one that is best explored in enactment over a series of several weeks.

When enacting Psyche, people often talk about how vulnerable she is to the whim of Aphrodite's jealousy, to the cheating oracle and to the envy of her sisters who upset her into mistrust. Psyche perhaps describes the state of the soul that, unless understood in its own terms, is seen to be weak in terms of world values. As in the story, the trials and testings of love, life and loss develop soul strength and a relationship with immortality.

The Queen Bee

This story of the kindly Simpleton who passes the tests and gets the Princess, while his clever brothers are turned to stone, has lots of dramatic potential. It is a good story to use with a fairly large group, needing scenes and atmospheres to be set, people to be ducks, bees and ants, and eventually the royal family and stone figures at the castle.

Rapunzel

A story that speaks to every age group, with a different resonance for every person taking part. In preparing for enactment, the tower without a door makes an evocative image for *bridging in*. This usually has to be improvised in some way. When Pat Watts brought Rapunzel to the training group, then working in a huge church hall with gas fires and cobwebs in its high windows, we were most lucky to discover an old, free-standing, circular stair, leading up to nowhere (probably, in its useful days, to a pulpit). Myth enactment doesn't rely on props, but those steps were a great gift. It's always worth looking out for site-specific props!

The Sacred Gift of Song, Dance and Festivity

Like *Akinidi and the Coming of Happiness*, this story is a model for dramatherapy and the healing joy of celebration. The heart image can be worked in *bridge in* and *bridge out* with a drum, indicating the beat of your heart before and after the story.

The Seal Woman

This is one of many stories from Scotland and Ireland in which seals can assume a human shape and people can turn into seals. Duncan Williamson, who collected seal stories on his travels around Scotland and put them into his books, disapproved of this particular story on the grounds that 'the Seal People do not take off their skins!' Our version was gathered from another, anonymous source in Scotland, becoming part of the Sesame repertoire for the simple reason that it works. Some practitioners like to work with the version by Clarissa Pinkola Estes, in her book *Women Who Run with the Wolves*, to which she gives the title 'Sealskin Soulskin'.[10]

The Snow Queen

Strictly speaking, *The Snow Queen* is not a myth or a fairytale, being a written story by a known author, though Hans Christian Anderson called his stories 'fairytales'. It has a linear shape. It is not, as traditional fairytales often are, held in a series of three events and a happily ever after. The story is long and, like the journey it describes, has a rather endless quality. For this reason, it needs extra careful containment in the form of strong warm-ups and *bridge ins* to hold the session together.

Working with clients, the splinter in the heart caused by the distorting mirror of the wicked goblin offers a resonant metaphor for low self-esteem and lack of confidence. We are not seeing ourselves aright. This image has successfully enabled many people in assertion training, rehabilitating after a stay in a psychiatric ward. When the glass splinter is removed, each person has the chance to spell ETERNITY from the ice flakes, being warmed into relationship with their own goodness pattern. (Sometimes the word 'eternity' can be interchanged for LOVE.)

---

10   Estes 1992.

A good *bridge in* for this story is mirroring. A can be the mover and B has the choice to mirror truthfully – or to playfully distort A's movement.

The Snow Queen was the story chosen for an enactment at Central School of Speech and Drama at which the pictures in the centre of this book were taken by Camilla Jessel Panufnik. The story was selected for that evening because of the time of year and the very frosty weather that had descended on London. People were cold.

The session plan used for this enactment is included before the colour picture section in the centre of the book.

After the session, participants were asked if the Snow Queen session had affected them. Four responses follow:

A – For me this session took me by surprise. I had no idea how powerful this fairytale could be. To me the session allowed me to reflect on the idea of love, letting go, sibling love and the idea of opposites. The cold and the warmth are two archetypal poles that affect all of us.

B – *The Snow Queen* is one of my favourite stories, not least because I played the narrator of the Snow Queen in a production at the Young Vic theatre. It was a difficult but extremely special experience at that time – light and dark, cold and warm. I was on the outside looking in, propelling the drama then. In the dramatherapy session, however, I was *in* the world of the story, which was a wonderful experience for me. I experienced 'an internal warmth' for days afterwards.

C – It meant I could experience yet another journey in comfort, with un-judgmental eyes watching. I was free, free at being me, although taking on the parts of others. It meant I gave parts of me that were then nurtured unconditionally and I received many pieces of puzzles which I held for others and these have left a positive imprint. I haven't a name or a full awareness of where this imprint is yet but it is definitely there.

D – Being in love and being left when the prince left me with the Snow Queen spoke to a lot of the losses in my life. But it was also good to have reparation in the story that may not have happened with my divorce. I loved the imagery around hot and cold and found the creativity of making the space with different props and bits of material really satisfying. As always the chance to let my body move itself in the warm-up exercises and do what it needs to do is great –

reminds me of the 5 Rhythms dancing I have done. Also I was able to express my feelings by using my body and not getting stuck in a heady wordy space.

The Star Woman

Probably the best known of all the Bushman stories, this one tells of a woman from the sky who marries a herdsman and tells him never to look in her basket. It was a favourite in the repertoire of the storyteller and writer Laurens Van der Post. Of the denouement, he said that, according to his Bushman source, the herdsman's unforgivable sin was not in disobeying his wife by looking in her basket, but in the fact that when he looked he could see nothing there.

This is the story for which Sesame's traditional *bridge in* consists of all participants becoming cows. For many people, being a cow is a wonderful experience. In our training group, this being cows went on for quite a while. The dusty church hall became a wide African plain. That scene, experienced and retained in the body as well as the imagination, has remained forever part of the story in our inner landscape. Earlier in this book (see Chapter 2) there is a reference to the great difficulty of de-roling people who have taken part in the story as cows.

Stone Soup

A trickster story with a great potential for humour that emerges naturally from serious, straightforward engagement in the process of soup making. It often brings up themes of who contributes what in a group and a sense of each person having something to bring to the whole.

The Story Bag

This is good story for encouraging people to think about telling their stories to each other.

A *bridge in* which can be fun and thought-provoking works in groups of threes or fours. After a warm-up where the group are working in sound rather than words:

A says 'Tell me the story about…'

She then makes up a 'gobbledygook' story (nonsense language).

B and C act this out as she tells it, responding to the affect and sound of what they hear. There is no logical comprehension required.

When stuck, B and C can ask A, 'How does the story go next?'

D interrupts, finding ways to prevent the story being told.

Swap roles, then discuss.

After the enactment, de-role and grounding, a final exercise goes round the circle:

Each person says: 'I am John, can you can hear me?'

The group members reply: 'Yes, John, we can hear you.'

The Tengu

This is a very short story that allows a lot of time and space for enjoyable warm-ups and *bridge ins*, making it particularly useful with new groups.

A Thorn in the King's Foot

Duncan Williamson (1928–2007), a great storyteller from the travelling people of Scotland, chose this wonder tale as the title story for his volume of Scottish tales for the Penguin Folklore Library, published in 1987.[11] Recorded and beautifully transcribed by Linda Williamson, his widow, Duncan's stories should be read in the vernacular for full enjoyment, especially as it is no longer possible to sit with him and hear them by the fire, or at a storytelling festival. Our version, like all the stories in the book, is pared down to essentials for enactment. Duncan was happy for it to be included in our collection, asserting as always that these traditional stories belong to everyone. He was always generous, encouraging his audience to tell the stories. This particular story works well for enactment, though it is long. Ideally, it should be given at least half a day or a full day, preparing the enactment in two parts.

Thousandfurs

A strong story that explores, among other things, the themes of incest and of individuation in relation to women. The Jungian analyst Marion Woodman has written about the story at some length, using its German title *Allerleirauh*, in her book *Leaving my Father's House: A Journey to*

---

11 Williamson 1987.

Conscious Femininity.[12] Marion's work with women, which focuses on eating disorders, is especially interesting to Sesame dramatherapists as she encourages her analysands to take part in workshops that explore physically, through dance movement, voice work and other art forms, themes that come up in their dreams and analytic sessions.

The Three Feathers

Very often we have to find ways to work with people who cannot move. This story is useful to work with as a seated story because the hero has to work from a fixed place.

The sessions can start with a simple game of imagining a present underneath your chair, which opens up the idea of reaching down rather than moving out into space.

The story also provides a means of thinking about descent at a lighter level than some of the bigger myths such as *Inanna in the Underworld* or *Chiron the Wounded Healer*.

Fun exercises with blowing a feather across the circle also introduce the theme playfully.

The Three Little Pigs

This story can work with people of all ages. Small children love to enact it straight. For adults, it is an enjoyable excuse for a romp and an excellent ice breaker.

Tiddalik the Frog

This story is much used in Sesame, particularly with children. It really amuses them. Sometimes it makes a connection with secrets and suppressed feelings. A child who has something he or she is keeping quiet about, but would dearly like to share with someone, will sometimes feel drawn to the part of Tiddalik. The enactment may then be followed by some kind of disclosure, the way Tiddalik lets out the water he has been keeping to himself. Tiddalik was brought into the dramatherapy repertoire by Alida Gersie, who included it in her collection *Earthtales: Storytelling in Times of Change*.[13]

---

12   Woodman 1992.
13   Gersie 1992.

The Twin Warrior Heroes

This Native American story was used very satisfactorily with a group of emotionally disturbed children because the hero role features twins. Often, children who were very competitive with each other were able to work well together on this journey to find the father.

The feather blessing of Spider Woman and the obstacles to be overcome bring two energies to the story. On one hand, the twin enactors have to be strong and wily, while at the same time they need to depend on 'magic' or other power. They have to remember the protection that has been given to them, which does not depend only on brain or brawn.

The story can also be used as an ending story for people leaving a situation, with the setting out of the twins seen as a parting from one way of being to make trails for the new. Exercises before can involve preparing to leave and considering the starting direction of the new journey.

Water Jar Boy, Childhood of the Human Hero

This story belongs to a Native American culture rooted in the concept of 'Circles of Life', in which myth is seen in terms of concentric circles, containing multiple layers of meaning that are added through the generations. The layers of meaning emerge at different stages in an individual's life. Cajete, writing about this traditional way of teaching and learning, describes how:

> Every myth has its concentric rings of meaning... The telling of a myth begins with a simple version for children, then moves to a slightly more complicated version for adolescents, to a deeper version for initiates, and to a still deeper version for the fully mature.[14]

Water Jar Boy is a beautiful example of such a myth, as the Sesame practitioner can discover through bringing it to different age groups for enactment!

Whisky Jack

There are few characters in this story, but it has beautiful potential for creating contrasting scenes, making the architectural shape of the great whale, the scene in its dark, slurping stomach, the birds pecking away

---

14   Cajete 1994, p.29.

the flesh and letting in the light, and the skeleton of the great fish drifting like a ship towards the shore.

This is a story that works well with instrumental music. An enactment with music can benefit from spending some time in the warm-up, experimenting with the percussion instruments and perhaps adding some vocal sound. A good way of introducing a group to the instruments, so that they discover that anyone can play them, is to invite each person to choose an instrument and sit with it in the circle. One person is invited to begin, making the sound of his or her chosen instrument, and the other instruments are added in, one by one round the circle. The key to success with this exercise is listening. If everyone listens, the result will be not cacophony but music. The exercise has been known to go on and on, like jazz. So it is as well to establish in advance that a signal will be given for the players to drop out, one by one round the circle, until it is silent. Otherwise, the exercise can seriously upset the timing of the enactment!

The White Snake

This story combines two familiar themes. The hero benefits from understanding the language of animals (as in Grimm's *The Three Languages*) and from his kindness to the creatures he meets, who come to his aid and help him to win a Princess (as in *The Queen Bee*). These themes come up frequently in Grimm's fairytales and seem to indicate something about living life in creative harmony with nature, as compared to going against nature, which invariably leads to trouble.

References

Bleek, W.H. and Lloyd, L.C. (1911) *Specimens of Bushman Folklore*. London: George Allen & Co.

Bly, R. (1990) *Iron John: A Book about Men*. Reading, MA: Addison-Wesley.

Blyton, E. (1939) *The Magic Faraway Tree*. London: Egmont Books.

Brook, P. (1968) *The Empty Space*. London: McGibbon & Kee.

Buuck, D. (2006) 'Ethnopoetics and Allegory.' Available at http://davidbuuck.com/downloads/criticism/ethnopoetics.pdf, accessed on 14 February 2013.

Cajete, G. (1994) *Look to the Mountain: An Ecology of Indigenous Education*. Durango, CO: Kivaki Press.

Caldecott, M. (1993) *Myths of the Sacred Tree*. Rochester, VT: Destiny Books.

Campbell, J. and Moyers, B. (1988) *The Power of Myth*. New York, NY: Doubleday.

Colum, P. (1944) *The Complete Grimm's Fairytales*. New York, NY: Pantheon.

Dekker, K. (1998) Paper for the Sesame Institute, London.

Edinger, E.F. (1972) *Ego and Archetype*. Boston, MA: Shambala.

Edinger, E.F. (1994) *The Eternal Drama: The Inner Meaning of Greek Mythology*. Boston, MA: Shambala.

Estes, C.P. (1992) 'Sealskin, Soulskin.' In C.P. Estes (ed.) *Women Who Run with the Wolves*, London: Rider.

Gersie, A. (1991) *Storymaking in Bereavement. Dragons Fight in the Meadow*. London: London: Jessica Kingsley Publishers.

Gersie, A. (1992) *Earthtales. Storytelling in Times of Change*. London: Merlin Press.

Gersie, A. (1996) *Dramatic Approaches to Brief Therapy*. London: Jessica Kingsley Publishers.

Gersie, A. and King, N. (1990) *Storymaking in Education and Therapy*. London: Jessica Kingsley Publishers.

Henderson, J. (1967) *Thresholds of Initiation*. Middletown, CT: Wesleyan University Press.

Hillman, J. (1965) *Suicide and the Soul*. Putnam, CT: Spring.

Hillman, J. (1983) *Inter Views*. New York, NY: Harper.

Hillman, J. (1997) *The Soul's Code*. New York: Bantam Books.

Johnson, D.R. (1994) 'Shame dynamics among creative arts therapists.' *The Arts in Psychotherapy 21*, 3, 173–178.

Jones, P. (1996) *Drama as Therapy. Theatre as Living*. London: Routledge.

Jung, C.G. (1956/1967) *Symbols of Transformation, CW5*. Princeton, NJ: Princeton University Press.

Jung C.G. (1968/1991) *The Archetypes and the Collective Unconscious, CW9, Part 1*. London: Routledge.

Jung, C.G. and Kerenyi, K. (1941) *The Science of Mythology*. Amsterdam: Pantheon.

Kearney, M. (1996) *Mortally Wounded: Stories of Soul Pain, Death and Healing*. Dublin: Marino.

Laban, R. (1980) *The Mastery of Movement* (Revised by Lisa Ullman). London: Macdonald and Evans.

Lewis, C.S. (1950) *The Lion, the Witch and the Wardrobe.* London, Macmillan.

Lindkvist, M.R. (1998) *Bring White Beads When You Call on the Healer.* New Orleans, LA: Rivendell House.

McGlashan, A. (1988) *The Savage and Beautiful Country.* Einsiedeln, Switzerland: Daimon Verlag.

Milne, A.A. (1928) *The House at Pooh Corner.* London: Methuen.

Ong, W. J. (1982) *Orality and Literacy,* London: Routledge.

Pearson, J. (1996) *Discovering the Self Through Drama and Movement: The Sesame Approach.* London: Jessica Kingsley Publishers.

Perera, S.B. (1981) *Descent to the Goddess: A Way of Initiation for Women.* Toronto, ON: Inner City Books.

Romanyshyn, R. (1999) *The Soul in Grief, Love, Death and Transformation.* Berkeley, CA: North Atlantic Books.

Romanyshyn, R. (2006) 'The wounded researcher: Levels of transference in the research process.' *Harvest: International Journal for Jungian Studies 52,* 1, 38–49.

Rowling, J.K. (1997–2007) *Harry Potter* series.

Scheub, H. (1998) *Story.* Madison: The University of Wisconsin Press.

Schrader, C. (2012) *Ritual Theatre.* London: Jessica Kingsley Publishers.

Slade, P. (1954) *Child Drama.* London: University of London Press.

Smail, M. (2004) *Sesame Newsletter, Spring 1994.* London: The Sesame Institute.

Travers, P.L. (1989) *What the Bee Knows.* London: Penguin Books.

Van der Post, L. (1993) Recording of a live storytelling session at the Temenos Academy, London.

Watts, P. (1992) 'Therapy in Drama.' In S. Jennings (ed.) *Dramatherapy Theory and Practice 2.* London: Routledge.

Watts, P. (1995) 'Working with Myth and Story.' In J. Pearson (ed.) *Discovering the Self Through Drama and Movement: The Sesame Approach.* London: Jessica Kingsley Publishers.

Williamson, D. (1987) *A Thorn in the King's Foot: Stories of the Scottish Travelling People.* London: Penguin.

Winnicott, D.W. (1960) 'The Theory of the Parent-Infant Relationship' and 'Ego Distortion in Terms of True and False Self.' In *The Maturational Processes and the Facilitating Environment.* London: Hogarth.

Winnicott, D.W. (1967) 'The Location of Cultural Experience.' In *Playing and Reality.* London: Tavistock Publications.

Wolkstein, D. and Kramer, S. (1983) *Inanna, Queen of Earth and Heaven.* New York, NY: Harper and Row.

Woodman, M. (1992) *Leaving My Father's House: A Journey to Conscious Femininity.* Boston, MA: Shambhala.

Zipes, J. (1995) *Creative Storytelling: Building Community, Changing Lives.* New York, NY: Routledge.

Further reading

Bettelheim, B. (1976) *The Uses of Enchantment: The Meaning and Importance of Fairy Tales.* London: Thames and Hudson.

Blackmer, J.D. (1989) *Acrobats of the Gods, Dance and Transformation.* Toronto: Inner City Books.

Campbell, J. (1949) *The Hero with a Thousand Faces.* New York, NY: Bollingen.

Campbell, J. (1972) *Myths to Live By.* New York, NY: Viking Press.

Eliade, M. (1957) *The Sacred and the Profane: The Nature of Religion.* Orlando, FL: Harcourt.

Johnson, R.A. (1993) *The Fisher King and the Handless Maiden: Understanding the Wounded Feeling Function in Masculine and Feminine Psychology.* New York, NY: HarperCollins.

Jung, E. and von Franz, M.-L. (1998) *The Grail Legend.* Princeton, NJ: Princeton University Press.

Levy-Strauss, C. (1978) *Myth and Meaning.* London: Routledge and Kegan Paul.

Luthi, M. (1970) *Once Upon a Time: On the Nature of Fairytales.* Bloomington, IN: University of Indiana.

Mellon, N. (1992) *Storytelling and the Art of Imagination.* Shaftesbury: Element.

Riordan, J. (1989) *The Sun Maiden and the Crescent Moon: Siberian Folk Tales.* Edinburgh: Cannongate.

Romanyshyn, R.D. (2007) *The Wounded Researcher.* New Orleans, LA: Spring.

Roose-Evans, J. (1994) *Passages of the Soul: Ritual Today.* London: Element.

Sawyer, R. (1942) *The Way of the Storyteller.* New York, NY: Viking.

Strenski, I. (ed.) (1993) *Malinowski and the Work of Myth.* Princeton, NJ: Princeton University Press.

Turner, V. (1982) *From Ritual to Theatre: The Human Seriousness of Play.* New York, NY: PAJ Publications.

Turner, V. (1987) *The Anthropology of Performance.* New York, NY: PAJ Publications.

Van Gennep, A. (1960) *The Rites of Passage.* London: Routledge.

Van der Post, L. (1965) *The Heart of the Hunter.* London: Hogarth.

Von Franz, M.-L. (1970) *The Interpretation of Fairytales.* Boston, MA: Shambhala.

Index